Vegetarian Recipe Book

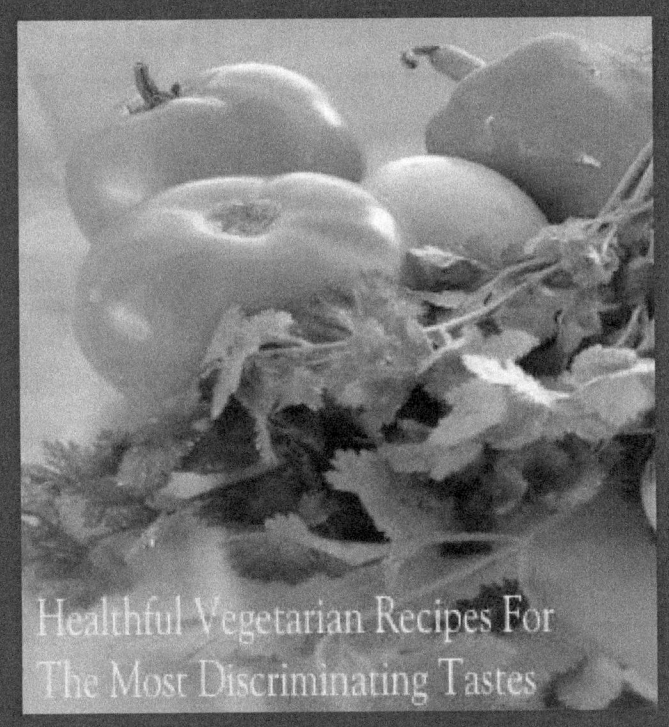

Vegetarian Recipe Book

Healthful Vegetarian Recipes For
The Most Discriminating Tastes

**Healthful Vegetarian Recipes For
The Most Discriminating Tastes.
This Recipe Book Contains over
1,000 Delicious Vegetarian Recipes!**

This ebook is brought to you by
NicheMarketingIdeas.Com.

SOUPS AND STEWS

ARTICHOKE SOUP.

1 lb. each of artichokes and potatoes, 1 Spanish onion, 1 oz. of butter, 1 pint of milk, and pepper and salt to taste. Peel, wash, and cut into dice the artichokes, potatoes, and onion. Cook them until tender in 1 quart of water with the butter and seasoning. When the vegetables are tender rub them through a sieve. Return the liquid to the saucepan, add the milk, and boil the soup up again. Add water if the soup is too thick. Serve with Allinson plain rusks, or small dice of bread fried crisp in butter or vege-butter.

HARICOT SOUP.

1 lb. of haricot beans, ½ lb. of onions, 1 lb. of turnips, 2 carrots, 2 sticks of celery, 1 teaspoonful of mixed herbs, ½ oz. of parsley, 1 oz. of butter, 2 quarts of water, pepper and salt to taste. Cut up the vegetables and set them to boil in the water with the haricot beans (which should have been steeped over night in cold water), adding the butter, herbs, and seasoning. Cook all very gently for 3-1/2 to 4 hours, stirring occasionally. When the beans are quite tender, rub the soup through a sieve, adding more water if needed; return it to the saucepan, add the parsley chopped up finely, boil it up and serve.

BARLEY SOUP.

8 oz. of pearl barley, 2 onions, 4 potatoes, ½ a teaspoonful of thyme, 1 dessertspoonful of finely chopped parsley, 3-1/2 pints of water, ½ pint of milk, 1 oz. of butter. Pick and wash the barley, chop up the onions, slice the potatoes. Boil the whole gently for 4 hours with the water, adding the butter, thyme, pepper and salt to taste. When the barley is quite soft, add the milk and parsley, boil the soup up, and serve.

BREAD SOUP.

½ lb. of stale crusts of Allinson wholemeal bread, 4 onions, 2 turnips, 1 stick of celery, 1 oz. of butter, ½ oz. of finely chopped parsley, 8 pints of water, ½ pint of milk. Soak the crusts in the water for 2 hours before they are put over the fire. Cut up into small dice the vegetables; add them to the bread with the butter and pepper and salt to taste. Allow all to simmer gently for 1 hour, then rub the soup through a sieve, return it to the saucepan, add the milk and parsley, and, if the flavour is liked, a little grated nutmeg; boil the soup up and serve at once.

CABBAGE SOUP.

1 fair-sized cabbage, a large Spanish onion, 1-1/2 oz. of butter, pepper and salt to taste, ½ saltspoonful of nutmeg, 1-1/2 pints of milk, 2 tablespoonfuls of Allinson fine wheatmeal. After preparing and washing the cabbage, shred up very fine, chop up the onion, set these two in a saucepan over the fire with 1 quart of water, the butter and seasoning, and let all cook gently for 1 hour, or longer it the vegetables are not quite tender. Add the milk and thickening when the vegetables are thoroughly tender, and let all simmer gently for 10 minutes; serve with little squares of toasted or fried bread, or Allinson plain rusks.

CABBAGE SOUP (French).

1 medium-sized cabbage, 1 lb. of potatoes, 1 oz. of butter, 3 pints of milk and water equal parts, pepper and salt to taste, 1 dessertspoonful of finely chopped parsley, and 2 blades of mace, and 1 dessertspoonful of Allinson fine wheatmeal. Wash the cabbage and shred it finely, peel the potatoes and cut them into small dice; boil the vegetables in the milk and water until quite tender, adding the mace, butter, and seasoning. When quite soft, rub the wheatmeal smooth with a little water, let it simmer with the soup for 5 minutes, add the parsley, and serve.

CAPER SOUP.

2 pints of water, 1 pint of milk, 1 large tablespoonful of capers, ½ lemon, 2 eggs, 1-1/2 oz. of Allinson fine wheatmeal, ½ oz. of butter, pepper and salt to taste. Boil the milk and water and butter, with seasoning to taste; thicken it with the wheatmeal rubbed smooth

with a little milk. Chop up the capers, add them and let the soup cook gently for 10 minutes; take it off the fire, beat up the eggs and add them carefully, that they may not curdle; at the last add the juice of the half lemon, re-heat the soup without allowing it to boil, and serve.

CARROT SOUP (1).

4 good-sized carrots, 1 head of celery, 1 onion, 3 oz. of Allinson wholemeal bread without crust, 1 oz. of butter, pepper and salt, and 1 blade of mace. Wash, scrape, and cut the carrots into dice. Prepare and cut up the onions and celery. Set the vegetables over the fire with 3 pints of water, adding the mace and seasoning. Let all cook until quite soft, which will probably be in 1-1/2 hours. If the carrots are old, they will take longer cooking. When the vegetables are tender, rub all through a sieve, return the soup to the saucepan, add the butter, allow it to boil up, and serve with sippets of toast.

CARROT SOUP (2).

4 good-sized carrots, 1 small head of celery, 1 fair-sized onion, 1 turnip, 3 oz. of breadcrumbs, 1-1/2 oz. of butter, 1 blade of mace, pepper and salt to taste. Scrape and wash the vegetables, and cut them up small; set them over the fire with 3 pints of water, the butter, bread, and mace. Let all boil together, until the vegetables are quite tender, and then rub them through a sieve. Return the mixture to the saucepan, season with pepper and salt, and if too thick add water to the soup, which should be as thick as cream, boil the soup up, and serve.

CAULIFLOWER SOUP.

1 medium-sized cauliflower, 1-1/2 pints of milk, 1 oz. of butter, 2 oz. of Allinson fine wheatmeal, pepper and salt to taste, a little nutmeg, and the juice of a lemon. Prepare the cauliflower by washing and breaking it into pieces, keeping the flowers whole, and boil in 1-1/2 pints of water, adding the butter, nutmeg, and seasoning. When the cauliflower is quite tender add the milk, boil it up, and thicken the soup with the wheatmeal, which should first be smoothed with a little cold water. Lastly, add the lemon juice, and serve the soup with sippets of toast.

CLEAR SOUP.

1 large Spanish onion, 1 teaspoonful of mixed herbs, ½ head of celery, 1-1/2 oz. butter, 1 carrot, 1 turnip, and pepper and salt to taste. Chop the onion up fine, and fry it brown in the butter, in the saucepan in which the soup is to be made, and add 5 pints of water. Prepare and cut into small pieces the carrot, turnip, and celery; add these, the nutmeg, herbs, and pepper and salt to the water, with the fried onions. When the vegetables are tender drain the liquid; return it to the saucepan, and boil the soup up.

CLEAR SOUP (with Dumplings).

2 large English onions, 1 teaspoonful of herbs, ½ teaspoonful of nutmeg, 1 carrot, 1 turnip, pepper and salt to taste, 1 oz. of butter, 3 pints of water. Chop up finely the onions and fry them brown in the butter in the saucepan in which the soup is to be made; add the water. Cut up in thin slices the carrot and turnip, add these, with the herbs, nutmeg, and seasoning to the soup. Let it boil for I hour, drain the liquid, return it to the saucepan, and when boiling add the dumplings prepared as follows: ½ pint of clear soup, 4 eggs, a little nutmeg, pepper and salt to taste. Beat the eggs well,

mix them with the soup, and season the mixture with nutmeg, pepper, and salt. Pour it into a buttered jug; set it in a pan with boiling water, and let the mixture thicken. Then cut off little lumps with a spoon, and throw these into the soup and boil up before serving.

CLEAR CELERY SOUP.

1 large head of celery or 2 small ones, 1 large Spanish onion, 2 oz. of butter, pepper and salt to taste, and 1 blade of mace. Chop the onion and fry it brown in the butter or Allinson vege-butter in the saucepan in which the soup is to be made. When brown, add 4 pints of water, the celery washed and cut into pieces, the mace, the pepper and salt. Let all cook until the celery is quite soft, then drain the liquid from the vegetables. Return it to the saucepan, boil the soup up, and add 1 oz. of vermicelli, sago, or Italian paste; let the soup cook until this is quite soft, and serve with sippets of crisp toast, or Allinson plain rusks.

COCOANUT SOUP.

2 cocoanuts grated, 2 blades of mace, 1 saltspoonful of cinnamon, 3 pints of water, the juice of a lemon, 2 eggs, 1 oz. of Allinson fine wheatmeal, pepper and salt to taste. Boil the cocoanut in the water, adding the mace, cinnamon, and seasoning. Let it cook gently for an hour; strain the mixture through a sieve and then return the soup to the saucepan. Make a paste of the eggs, wheatmeal, and lemon juice, add it to the soup and let it boil up before serving; let it simmer for 5 minutes, and serve with a little plain boiled rice.

CORN SOUP.

1 breakfastcupful of fresh wheat, 1 quart of water, ½ pint of milk, ½ oz. of butter, ½ oz. of finely chopped parsley, 1 oz. of eschalots,

seasoning to taste. Steep the wheat over night in the water and boil it in the same water for 3 hours, add the butter, the eschalots, chopped up very fine, and pepper and salt. Let the whole simmer very gently for another ½ hour, add the milk and parsley, boil the soup up once more, and serve.

LEEK SOUP (1).

2 bunches of leeks, 1-1/2 pints of milk, 1 oz. of butter, 1 lb. of potatoes, pepper and salt to taste, and the juice of a lemon. Cut off the coarse part of the green ends of the leeks, and cut the leeks lengthways, so as to be able to brush out the grit. Wash the leeks well, and see no grit remains, then cut them in short pieces. Peel, wash, and cut up the potatoes, then cook both vegetables with 2 pints of water. When the vegetables are quite tender, rub them through a sieve. Return the mixture to the saucepan, add the butter, milk, and seasoning, and boil the soup up again. Before serving add the lemon juice; serve with sippets of toast.

LEEK SOUP (2).

1 dozen leeks, 1-1/2 pints of milk, 1 lb. of potatoes, 1 oz. of butter, pepper and salt to taste, and the juice of a lemon (this last may be omitted if not liked). Prepare the leeks as in the previous recipe, cut them into pieces about an inch long. Peel and wash the potatoes and cut them into dice. Set the vegetables over the fire with 1 quart of water, and cook them until tender, which will be in about 1 hour. When soft rub all through a sieve and return the soup to the saucepan. Add the milk, butter, and seasoning, boil up, and add the lemon juice just before serving. Should the soup be too thick add a little hot water. Serve with Allinson plain rusks.

LENTIL SOUP.

1 lb. each of lentils and potatoes, 1 large Spanish onion, 1 medium-sized head of celery (or the outer pieces of a head of celery, saving the heart for table use), 1 breakfastcupful of tinned tomatoes or ½ lb. of fresh ones, 1 oz. of butter, pepper and salt to taste. Chop the onion up roughly, and fry it in the butter until beginning to brown. Pick and wash the lentils, and set them over the fire with 2 quarts of water or vegetable stock, adding the fried onion. Peel, wash, and cut up the potatoes, prepare the celery, cut it into small pieces, and add all to the lentils. When they are nearly soft add the tomatoes. When all the ingredients are quite tender rub them through a sieve. Return the soup to the saucepan, add pepper and salt, and more water if the soup is too thick. Serve with sippets of toast.

MACARONI STEW.

6 oz. of cold boiled macaroni, 1 large Spanish onion, 1 carrot, ½ lb. of tomatoes, ¼ lb. of mushrooms, 2 oz. of grated cheese, 1 oz. of butter, pepper and salt to taste. Wash, prepare, and cut up the vegetables in small pieces. Cover them with water and stew them until tender, adding the butter and seasoning. When tender add the macaroni cut into finger lengths, and the cheese.

MILK SOUP.

2 onions, 2 turnips, 1 head of celery, 3 pints of milk, 1 pint of water, 2 tablespoonfuls of Allinson fine wheatmeal, pepper and salt to taste. Chop up the vegetables and boil them in the water until quite tender. Rub them through a sieve, return the whole to the saucepan, add pepper and salt, rub the wheatmeal smooth in the milk, let the soup simmer for 5 minutes, and serve.

MILK SOUP (suitable for Children).

1-1/2 pints of milk, 1 egg, 1 tablespoonful of Allinson fine wheatmeal, 1-1/2 oz. of sultanas, sugar to taste. Boil 1-1/4 pints of milk, add the sugar, beat up the egg with the rest of the milk and mix the wheatmeal smooth with it; stir this into the boiling milk, add the sultanas, and let the soup simmer for 10 minutes.

OATMEAL SOUP.

6 oz. of coarse oatmeal, the outer part of a head of celery, 1 Spanish onion, 1 turnip, 1 oz. of butter, and pepper and salt. Wash and cut the vegetables up small, set them over the fire with 2 quarts of water. When boiling, stir in the oatmeal and allow all to cook gently for 2 hours. Rub the mixture well through a sieve, adding hot water it necessary. Return the soup to the saucepan, add the butter and pepper and salt, and let it boil up. The soup should be of a smooth, creamy consistency. Serve with sippets of toast or Allinson plain rusks.

ONION SOUP (French).

½ lb. onions, 3 oz. grated cheese, 2 oz. butter, some squares of Allinson wholemeal bread, pepper and salt to taste. Peel and chop the onions, and fry them a nice brown in the butter. When brown add to it the cheese and 3 pints of water. Boil all up together and season to taste. Place the bread in the tureen, pour the boiling soup over it, and serve.

PARSNIP SOUP.

3 parsnips, 1 onion, 1 head of celery, ½ oz. of butter, ½ pint of milk, 1 quart of water, 1 tablespoonful of Allinson fine wheatmeal, 1 tablespoonful of vinegar, pepper and salt. Scrape the parsnips and cut them up finely, cut up the celery and onion, and set the

vegetables over the fire with the water, butter, and pepper and salt to taste: when they are quite tender rub them through a sieve. Return the soup to the saucepan, add the milk and the thickening, boil up for five minutes, and before serving add the vinegar. This latter may be left out if preferred.

PEA SOUP.

1 lb. of split peas, 1 lb. of potatoes, peeled, washed, and cut into pieces, 1 Spanish onion, 1 carrot, 1 turnip, ½ head of celery or a whole small one, 1 oz. of butter, pepper and salt to taste, Pick and wash the peas, and set them to boil in 2 quarts of water. Add the potatoes and the other vegetables, previously prepared and cut into small pieces, the butter and seasoning. When all the ingredients are soft, rub them through a sieve and return them to the saucepan. If the soup is too thick, add more water. Boil it up, and serve with fresh chopped mint, or fried dice of Allinson wholemeal bread. Allow 3 to 4 hours for the soup.

PEASE BROSE.

This is made by the Scottish peasant in this way. He puts some pea flour into a basin, and pours boiling water over it, at the same time stirring and thoroughly mixing the meal and water together. When mixed he adds a little salt, pepper, and butter, and eats it with or without oatcake.

PORTUGUESE SOUP.

4 onions, 4 tomatoes, 1 oz. of grated cheese, ¼ lb. of stale Allinson wholemeal bread, 1 quart of water, 1 oz. of butter, 1 even teaspoonful of herbs, pepper and salt to taste. Slice the onions and fry them until brown, add the tomatoes skinned and sliced, the water, herbs, and pepper and salt, and let the whole

boil gently for 1 hour. Cut up the bread into dice, and put it into the tureen, pour the soup over it, cover, and let it stand for 10 minutes to allow the bread to soak; sprinkle the cheese over before serving.

POTATO SOUP.

2 lbs. of potatoes, ½ stick of celery or the outer stalks of a head of celery, saving the heart for table use; 1 large Spanish onion, 1 pint of milk, 1 oz. of butter, a heaped up tablespoonful of finely chopped parsley, and pepper and salt to taste. Peel, wash, and cut in pieces the potatoes, peel and chop roughly the onion, prepare and cut in small pieces the celery. Cook the vegetables in three pints of water until they are quite soft. Rub them through a sieve, return the fluid mixture to the saucepan; add the milk, butter, and seasoning, and boil the soup up again; if too thick add more water. Mix the parsley in the soup just before serving.

RICE SOUP.

3 oz. of rice, 4 oz. of grated cheese, a breakfastcupful of tomato juice, 1 oz. of butter, pepper and salt to taste. Boil the rice till tender in 2-1/2 pints of water, with the butter and seasoning. When quite soft, add the tomato juice and the cheese; stir until the soup boils and the cheese is dissolved, and serve. If too much of the water has boiled away, add a little more.

RICE AND GREEN-PEA SOUP.

2 oz. of rice, 1 breakfastcupful of shelled green peas, 1 pint of milk, 1 quart of water, 1 oz. of butter. Boil the rice in the water for 10 minutes, add the peas, the butter and pepper and salt to taste. Let it cook until the rice and

peas are tender, add the milk and boil the soup up before serving.

RICE AND ONION SOUP.

4 onions, 3 oz. of rice, 1-1/2 oz. of butter, 3 pints of water, pepper and salt. Chop the onions up very finely, and fry them with the butter until slightly browned; add the rice, seasoning, and water, and let the whole cook gently until quite soft. A tablespoonful of finely chopped parsley may be added.

ST. ANDREW'S SOUP.

4 large potatoes, 1 pint of clear tomato juice (from tinned tomatoes), 1 pint of milk, 1 pint of water, 2 eggs, 1 oz. of butter, seasoning to taste. Boil the potatoes in their skins; when tender peel and pass them through a potato masher. Put the potatoes into a saucepan with the butter, tomato juice, and water, adding pepper and salt to taste. Allow the soup to simmer for 10 minutes, then add the milk; boil up again, remove the saucepan to the cool side of the stove and stir in the eggs well beaten. Serve at once with sippets of toast, or Allinson plain rusks.

SCARLET RUNNER SOUP.

1-1/2 lbs. of French beans or scarlet runners, 1 onion, 1 carrot, 1 stick of celery, ½ oz. of butter, 1 teaspoonful of thyme, 2 quarts of water, pepper and salt to taste, and 2 oz. of Allinson fine wheatmeal. String the beans and break them up in small pieces, cut up the other vegetables and add them to the water, which should be boiling; add also the butter and pepper and salt. Allow all to cook until thoroughly tender, then rub through a sieve. Return the soup to the saucepan (adding more water if it has boiled away much), and thicken it with the wheatmeal; let it simmer for 5 minutes, and serve with fried sippets of bread.

SORREL SOUP (1).

½ lb. of sorrel, 1-1/2 lbs. of potatoes, 1 oz. of butter, pepper and salt, 3 pints of water. Pick, wash, and chop fine the sorrel, peel and cut up in slices the potatoes, and set both over the fire with the water, butter, and seasoning to taste; when the potatoes are quite tender, pass the soup through a sieve. Serve with sippets of toast.

SORREL SOUP (2).

1 lb. of sorrel, 1 large Spanish onion, 3 pints of water, 1 oz. of butter, pepper and salt to taste, ½ lb. of Allinson wholemeal bread cut into small dice. Pick, wash, and chop up the sorrel, chop up the onion, and boil both with the water, butter, pepper, and salt until the onion is quite tender. Place the bread in the soup-tureen and pour the soup over it. Cover it up, and let the bread soak for a few minutes before serving.

SORREL SOUP (French) (3).

1 lb. of sorrel, 1 oz. of butter, 2 tablespoonfuls of Allinson fine wheatmeal, 2 quarts of water, pepper and salt, 2 eggs. Pick and wash the sorrel and drain the water. Set it over the fire with the butter and stew for 5 minutes, add the wheatmeal, and stir it with the sorrel for 5 minutes; add the water, pepper and salt to taste, and let the soup simmer for ½ an hour; before serving add the eggs well beaten, but do not allow them to boil, as this would make them curdle; serve with sippets of toast.

SPANISH SOUP.

3 pints of chestnuts peeled and skinned, 2 Spanish onions, 6 potatoes, 2 turnips cut up in dice, 1 teaspoonful of thyme, 1 dessertspoonful of vinegar, 2 oz. of grated cheese, 1 oz. of butter, 2 quarts of water, pepper and salt to taste. Boil the chestnuts and vegetables gently until quite tender, which will take 1-1/2 hours. Rub them through a sieve and return the soup to the saucepan; add the butter; vinegar, and pepper and salt to taste. Let it boil 10 minutes, and sift in the cheese before serving.

SPINACH SOUP.

2 lbs. of spinach, 1 chopped up onion, 1 oz. of butter, 1 pint of milk, the juice of 1 lemon, 1-1/2 oz. of Allinson fine wheatmeal, and pepper and salt to taste. This will make about 3 pints of soup. Wash the spinach well, and cook it in 1 pint of water with the onion and seasoning. When the spinach is quite soft, rub all through a sieve. Mix the wheatmeal with the melted butter as in the previous recipe, stir into it the spinach, add the milk; boil all up, and add the lemon juice last of all. If the soup is too thick, add a little water.

SPRING SOUP.

2 carrots, 1 turnip, ½ head celery, 10 small spring onions, 1 tea-cup of cauliflower cut into little branches, heart of small white cabbage lettuce, small handful of sorrel, 1 leaf each of chervil and of tarragon, ¼ pint of peas, ¼ pint asparagus points, ¼ pint croutons, 1 quart of water. Cut the carrots and turnip into small rounds, or to shape; add them with the chopped-up celery, whole onions, and cauliflower, to a quart of water, and bring to the boil; simmer for ½ an hour. Stamp the sorrel and lettuce into small round pieces, and add them with the leaf of chervil and tarragon to the soup, together with 1 teaspoonful of

sugar. When all is quite tender add the peas and asparagus points, freshly cooked; serve with croutons.

SUMMER SOUP.

1 cucumber, 2 cabbage lettuces, 1 onion, small handful of spinach, a piece of mint, 1 pint shelled peas, 2 oz. butter. Wash and cut up the lettuces, also cut up the cucumber and onion, put them into a stewpan, together with ½ pint of peas, the mint, and butter. Cover with about 1 quart of cold water, bring to the boil, and simmer gently for 3 hours. Then strain off the liquid and pass the vegetables through a sieve. Add them to the liquid again, and set on the fire. Season and add ½ pint green peas previously boiled.

TAPIOCA AND TOMATO SOUP.

2 oz. of tapioca, 1 lb. of tomatoes, 1 carrot, 1 turnip, 1 teaspoonful of herbs, 1 blade of mace, 1 oz. of butter, pepper and salt to taste, and 3 pints of water. Peel, wash, and cut up finely the vegetables and stew them in the butter for 10 minutes. Add the water, the tomatoes skinned and cut in slices, the herbs and seasoning to taste; when the soup is boiling, sprinkle in the tapioca, let all cook until quite tender, pass the soup through a sieve, return it to the saucepan, and boil it up before serving.

TOMATO SOUP (1).

1-1/2 lbs. of tomatoes (or 1 tin of tomatoes), 1 oz. of butter, 3 pints of water (only 2 if tinned tomatoes are used), 2 oz. of rice, 1 large onion, 1 teaspoonful of herbs, pepper and salt to taste. Cut the tomatoes into slices, chop fine the onion, and let them cook with the water for about 20 minutes. Strain the mixture, return the liquid to the saucepan, and add the other ingredients and seasoning. Let the soup cook gently until the rice is tender.

TOMATO SOUP (2).

1 tin of tomatoes, or 2 lbs. of fresh ones, 1 large Spanish onion or 2 small ones, 2 oz. of butter, pepper and salt to taste, 1 oz. vermicelli, and 2 bay leaves (these may be left out it desired). Peel the onion and chop it up roughly. Fry it brown with the butter in the saucepan in which the soup should be made. When the onion is browned add the tomatoes (the fresh ones should be sliced), the bay leaves and 3 pints of water; let all cook together for ½ an hour. Then drain the liquid through a strainer or sieve without rubbing anything through; return the soup to the saucepan, add seasoning and the vermicelli, and allow the soup to cook until the vermicelli is soft, which will take from 5 to 10 minutes.

VEGETABLE SOUP.

2 large turnips, 2 large carrots, 2 Spanish onions, 1 teacupful of pearl barley, 1-1/2 oz. butter, ½ pint of milk, salt and pepper to taste. Cover the vegetables with cold water and allow them to boil from 2 to 3 hours, then rub through a sieve and add butter and milk. It too thick, add more milk. Boil up and serve.

VEGETABLE MARROW SOUP.

1 medium-sized marrow, 1 onion, ½ oz. of finely chopped parsley, 2 tablespoonfuls of Allinson fine wheatmeal, 1 pint of milk, 1 quart of water, ½ oz. of butter, pepper and salt to taste. Remove the pips from the marrow, cut it into pieces, chop up fine the onions, and cook the vegetables for 20 minutes, adding the butter, pepper, and salt. Rub through a sieve, return the soup to the saucepan, rub the fine wheatmeal smooth with the milk, add this to

the soup, allow it to simmer for 5 minutes, and add the parsley before serving.

WHITE SOUP.

4 oz. of ground almonds, 1 pint of milk, 1 pint of water, 1 oz. of vermicelli, 2 blades of mace, pepper and salt. Let the almonds and mace simmer in the water and milk for ½ of an hour, remove the mace, add pepper and salt to taste, and the vermicelli. Let the soup cook gently until the vermicelli is soft, and serve.

BATTERS

These dishes take the place of omelets and frequently of pies, to both of which they are in many particulars similar. The batter is used to keep the ingredients together, and adds to their wholesomeness.

BATTER CELERY.

1 large head of celery, 1 pint of milk, 3 eggs, 6 oz. Allinson fine wheatmeal, 2 oz. butter, 1 English onion, pepper and salt to taste. Prepare the celery, cut it into small pieces, chop up the onion pretty fine, and stew both gently in half the milk and the butter and seasoning. Make a batter meanwhile with the rest of the milk, the eggs and the wheatmeal. When the celery and onion are quite tender mix the batter with them; grease a pie-dish, pour the mixture into it, and bake the savoury for 1-1/2 hours. Eat with potatoes and tomato sauce.

BATTER POTATO.

1-1/2 lbs. of potatoes, two good-sized English onions, 1 pint of milk, ½ lb. of Allinson fine wheatmeal, 3 eggs, 2-1/2 oz. of butter, pepper and salt to taste. Peel and wash the potatoes, and slice them ¼ inch thick, then dry them on a cloth. Chop fine the onions. Put the butter into the frying-pan, and let it get boiling hot, turn into it the potatoes and onions, and fry them together, stirring frequently until the vegetables begin to brown and get soft. Make a batter of the milk, meal, and eggs, stir the fried potatoes and onions into it, and season with pepper and salt. Grease a pie-dish, turn the mixture into it, and bake the savoury for 1-1/2 hours. Serve with vegetables and tomato sauce. This is a very tasty dish.

BATTER VEGETABLE.

½ lb. of turnips, ½ lb. of carrots, ½ lb. of potatoes, ½ lb. of shelled green peas (if in season), ½ lb. of onions, 8 oz. of Allinson fine wheatmeal, 1 pint of milk, 3 eggs, 2 oz. of butter, pepper and salt. Cut the vegetables into small dice; fry them in the butter until fairly well cooked. Make the batter with the milk, wheatmeal, and the eggs well beaten; add the vegetables and seasoning. Bake the mixture in a pie-dish for 1-1/2 hours in a moderate oven.

SAVOURIES

ARTICHOKES AUX TOMATOES.

2 lbs. of artichokes, 1-1/2 lbs. of tomatoes (or three parts of a tin of tomatoes), 1 oz. of Allinson fine wholemeal, 1 oz. of butter, pepper and salt to taste, ½ dozen eschalots. Parboil the artichokes, drain them, and cut them into slices. Make tomato sauce as follows: Chop the eschalots up very finely, slice the tomatoes and stew both in ¾ pint of water for 20 minutes, adding seasoning and the butter; thicken the sauce with the wheatmeal, rub

through a sieve, pour it over the artichokes and stew both gently until the artichokes are quite tender; serve with potatoes.

BEAN PIE.

This is made from boiled beans, which are put in a pie-dish, soaked tapioca, flavouring herbs, pepper, salt, and butter are added, a cup of water is poured in to make the gravy, a crust is put on the top, and then baked for 1 hour or so. This is a tasty dish. Cold beans are very nice if warmed in a frying-pan with oil or butter, and may be eaten with potatoes, vegetables, and sauce. Mashed beans, flavoured with pepper, salt, and mace, and put into pots make an excellent substitute for potted meat.

BREAD AND CHEESE SAVOURY.

½ lb. of Allinson wholemeal bread, 3 oz. of grated cheese, 1 pint of milk, 3 eggs, pepper and salt to taste, a little nutmeg, and some butter. Cut the bread into slices and butter them: arrange in layers in a pie-dish, spreading some cheese between the layers, and dusting with pepper, salt, and a little nutmeg. Finish with a good sprinkling of cheese. Whip up the eggs, mix them with the milk and pour the mixture over the bread and cheese in the pie-dish. Pour the custard back into the basin, and repeat the pouring over the contents of the pie-dish. If this is done 2 or 3 times the top slices of bread and butter get soaked and then bake better. This should also be done when a bread and butter pudding is made. Bake the savoury until brown, which it will be in about ¾ of an hour.

BUTTER BEANS WITH PARSLEY SAUCE.

Pick the beans, wash them, and steep them over night in boiling water, just covering them.

Allow 2 or 3 oz. of beans for each person. In the morning, let them cook gently in the water they are steeped in with the addition of a little butter, until quite soft, which will be in about 2 hours. The beans should be cooked in only enough water to keep them from burning, therefore, when it boils away, add only just sufficient for absorption. The sauce is made thus: 1 pint of milk, 1 tablespoonful of Allinson fine wheatmeal, a handful of finely chopped parsley, the juice of ½ a lemon, pepper and salt to taste. Boil the milk and thicken it with the flour, which should first be smoothed with a little cold milk, then last of all add the lemon juice, the seasoning, and the parsley. This dish should be eaten with potatoes and green vegetables.

CARROTS AND RICE.

1 breakfastcupful of rice, 6 medium-sized carrots, 2 oz. of butter, 1 tablespoonful of finely chopped Parsley, 1 tablespoonful of Allinson fine wheatmeal, pepper and salt to taste. Boil the rice in 1 quart of water until quite tender and dry; meanwhile slice the carrots and stew them in 1 pint of water and 1 oz. of butter until quite tender, thicken them with the meal, add seasoning and the parsley. Set the rice in the form of a ring on a dish, pile the carrots in the centre, sprinkle a few breadcrumbs over the whole, also the butter cut into little bits, and bake the dish in a moderate oven for 20 minutes.

CAULIFLOWER AND POTATO PIE.

1 fair-sized boiled (cold) cauliflower, 1 lb. of cold boiled potatoes, 1 pint of milk, 3 eggs, 8 oz. of Allinson fine wheatmeal, 1-1/2 oz. of butter, 4 oz. of grated cheese, pepper and salt to taste. Cut up the cauliflower and potatoes, sprinkle half the cheese between the vegetables, make a batter of the milk and eggs

and meal, add seasoning to it, place the vegetables in a pie-dish, pour the batter over them, cut the butter into little bits and put them on the top of the pie, sprinkle the rest of the cheese over all, and bake for 1 hour.

CAULIFLOWER PIE.

1 small cauliflower, ¾ lb. of potatoes, ½ lb. of Allinson fine wheatmeal, 3 eggs, ¾ pint of milk, 1 oz. of butter, 1 saltspoonful of nutmeg, pepper and salt. Parboil the cauliflower and potatoes, cut the former into pieces and slice the potatoes; place both in a pie-dish with the butter and seasoning; make a batter of the meal, milk, and the eggs, well beaten; pour it over the vegetables, mix well, and bake 1-1/2 hours.

CELERY À LA PARMESAN.

2 heads of celery, 1 pint of milk, 2 oz. of Parmesan, or any other cooking cheese, 2 tablespoonfuls of breadcrumbs, 1 oz. of butter. Cut the celery into pieces 3 inches long, stew it in the milk until tender; drain the milk and make a sauce of it, thickening with Allinson fine wheatmeal, and adding the cheese and seasoning to taste. Put the celery into a pie-dish, pour the sauce over it, sprinkle the breadcrumbs over the whole, place the butter in little pieces on the top, and bake for 15 minutes in a moderate oven.

CELERY CROQUETTES.

1 or 2 heads of celery, a teacupful of dried and sifted Allinson breadcrumbs, 2 eggs, pepper and salt to taste. Well wash the celery, remove the coarse outer stalks, and steam the parts used until they are a little tender. Then cut them into pieces about 2 inches long, dip them first into the egg whipped up, then into the breadcrumbs, and fry them in boiling butter,

vege-butter, or olive oil until a nice brown; dust with pepper and salt, and serve up very hot; eat with white or tomato sauce.

CHESTNUT PIE.

2 lbs. of chestnuts, 1 head of celery, 1 large Spanish onion, ½ lb. of Allinson fine wheatmeal, 4 oz. of butter, pepper and salt. Boil the chestnuts until partly tender, and remove the skins; cut the celery into pieces, removing the outer very hard pieces only, slice the onion and stew until tender in 1 pint of water; mix all the ingredients together, adding 1 oz. of the butter and seasoning to taste; make some pastry of the meal, 3 oz. of butter, and a little cold water; turn the vegetables into a pie-dish, cover the dish with the pastry, and bake the pie for 1 hour; serve with brown gravy.

COLCANON.

1 large cabbage, 1 pint of mashed potatoes, 2 oz. of grated cheese, 2 eggs, 1 oz. of butter, ½ saltspoonful of nutmeg, pepper and salt to taste. Boil the cabbage in 1 pint of water until quite tender, drain the water off to keep for stock, chop the cabbage up fine; mix it with the mashed potatoes, the butter and seasoning and the grated cheese; beat up the eggs, and mix these well with the rest; press the mixture into a greased mould, heat all well through in the oven or in a steamer, turn out and serve with a white sauce. This can be made from cold potatoes and cold cabbage.

CORN PUDDING.

1 tin of sweet corn, 1 pint of milk, 4 eggs, 1 oz. of butter, 8 oz. of Allinson fine wheatmeal, ½ saltspoonful of nutmeg, pepper and salt to taste. Make a batter of the meal, eggs and

milk, add the other ingredients, pour the mixture into a pie-dish, and let it bake 1 hour.

CURRY BALLS.

8 oz. of rice, ½ oz. of butter, 1 good teaspoonful of curry, 2 eggs, pepper and salt to taste, some oil or butter for frying, and 1 teacupful of raspings. Boil the rice in 1 pint of water, adding the butter and seasoning. When the rice is dry and tender mix in the curry, beat up 1 egg, and bind the rice with that. Form into balls, dip them in the other egg, well beaten, then into the raspings and fry them a nice brown in oil or vege-butter.

CURRY SAVOURY.

1 breakfastcupful of rice, 1 ditto of Egyptian lentils, 1 lb. of tomatoes, 1 dessertspoonful of curry, 2 eggs well beaten, 1 oz. of butter, salt to taste. Boil the rice and lentils together until quite tender, and let them cool a little. Slice the tomatoes into a pie-dish, mix the curry, eggs, and salt with the rice and lentils, add a little milk it necessary; spread the mixture over the tomatoes, with the butter in bits over the top, and bake the savoury from ½ to 1 hour.

FAVOURITE PIE.

3 oz. of macaroni, 2 breakfastcupfuls of Allinson breadcrumbs, 2 onions, chopped very fine, 2 breakfastcupfuls of tinned tomatoes, 3 eggs, well beaten, 3 oz. of butter, 1 dessertspoonful of curry, salt to taste. Boil the macaroni until tender, and cut it up into pieces 1 inch long; fry the onion brown in the butter, mix the breadcrumbs with the tomatoes, add the eggs, curry, onion and salt, and mix all this with the macaroni; turn the mixture into a pie-dish, and bake the pie for 1 hour.

FORCEMEAT BALLS.

2 oz. of breadcrumbs, 6 oz. of boiled and grated potatoes, 1 gill of milk, 2 eggs, some Allinson fine wheatmeal ¼ teaspoonful of nutmeg, 3 finely chopped onions, 2 handfuls of spinach, 1 handful of parsley, 1 ditto of lettuce, all chopped fine. Soak the breadcrumbs in the milk, add the potatoes, eggs well beaten, all the vegetables and seasoning; mix sufficient of the wheatmeal with the rest to make the mixture into a fairly firm paste, form this into balls, drop these in boiling clear soup or water (according to requirements), and boil them for 5 to 10 minutes.

HAGGIS.

2 oz. of wheatmeal, 1 oz. of rolled oatmeal, 1 egg, ½ oz. of oiled butter, ½ lb. small sago, 3 eggs, 1 large Spanish onion, 1 dessertspoonful of mixed powdered herbs, 1 oz. of butter, pepper and salt to taste, and a little milk if needed. Swell the sago over the fire with as much water as it will absorb; when quite soft put into it the butter to melt, and, when melted, mix in the oatmeal and wheatmeal. Grate the onion, and whip up the eggs; mix all the ingredients together, not forgetting the herbs and seasoning. The whole should be a thick porridgy mass; if too dry add a little milk. Butter a pudding basin, pour into it the mixture, place a piece of buttered paper over it, tie a pudding cloth over the basin, and steam the haggis for 3 hours.

HERB PIE.

1 handful of parsley, 1 handful of spinach, and 1 of mustard and cress, 2 lettuce hearts sliced fine, 2 small onions, and a little butter, 3 eggs, 1 pint of milk, and ½ lb. of Allinson fine wheatmeal. Chop all the vegetables up finely, and mix them with a batter made of the milk,

meal, and eggs; season it with pepper and salt; mix well; pour the mixture into a buttered pie-dish, place bits of butter over the top, and bake it for 1-1/2 hours.

HOT-POT.

2 lbs. of potatoes, ¾ lb. of onions, 1 breakfastcupful of tinned tomatoes, or ½ lb. of sliced fresh ones, 1 teaspoonful of thyme, 1-1/2 oz. butter, pepper and salt to taste. Those who do not like tomatoes can leave them out, and the dish will still be very savoury. The potatoes should be peeled, washed, and cut into thin slices, and the onions peeled and cut into thin slices. Arrange the vegetables and tomatoes in layers; dust a little pepper and salt between the layers, and finish with a layer of potatoes. Cut the butter into little bits, place them on the top of the potatoes, fill the dish with hot water, and bake the hot-pot for 2 hours or more in a hot oven. Add a little more hot water if necessary while baking to make up for what is lost in the cooking.

LEEK PIE.

1 bunch of leeks, 1 lb. of potatoes, ½ teaspoonful of herbs, a little nutmeg, 1 pint of milk, pepper and salt to taste, 8 oz. of Allinson fine wheatmeal, 3 eggs, 1 oz. of butter. Cut up into dice the potatoes and leeks, parboil them in 1 pint of water, adding the herbs, butter, and seasoning; place the vegetables in a pie-dish, make a batter with the milk, eggs, and meal, pour it over the vegetables, mix all well, and bake the pie 1-1/2 to 2 hours in a moderate oven.

LENTIL PIE.

½ lb. of lentils, 1 lb. of potatoes, 1 lb. of tomatoes, 1 Spanish onion, 1 heaped-up teaspoonful of herbs, 3 hard-boiled eggs, 1-1/2 oz. of butter, pepper and salt to taste. Have the lentils cooked beforehand. Peel, wash, and cut into dice the potatoes and onion, and fry them in the butter until nearly soft. Scald and slice the tomatoes, and mix the fried vegetables, lentils, tomatoes, herbs, and seasoning well together. Turn the mixture into a pie-dish, and pour over as much water or vegetable stock as may be required for gravy. Quarter the eggs and place them on the top. Cover with a short crust, and bake the pie for 1 to 1-1/2 hours.

LENTIL RISSOLES.

½ lb. of lentils, 1 finely chopped onion, 1 breakfastcupful of breadcrumbs, 1 breakfastcupful of tinned tomatoes, 1-1/2 oz. of butter, 2 eggs, pepper and salt to taste, some raspings, butter, vege-butter or oil for frying. Pick and wash the lentils, and boil them in enough water to cover them; when this is absorbed add the tomatoes, and if necessary gradually a little more water to prevent the lentils from burning. Fry the onion in 1-1/2 oz. of butter, mix it with the lentils as they are stewing, and add pepper and salt to taste. When the lentils are quite soft, and like a pureé (which will take from 1 to 1-1/2 hours), set them aside to cool. Mix the lentils and the breadcrumbs, beat up one of the eggs and add it to the mixture, beating all well together. If it is too dry, add a very little milk, but only just enough to make the mixture keep together. Form into rissoles, beat up the second egg, roll them into the egg and raspings, and fry the rissoles a nice brown in boiling butter or oil. Drain and serve.

LENTIL TURNOVERS.

6 oz. of lentils, 6 oz. of mushrooms, 1 English onion chopped very fine, 1 ounce of butter, 1 dessertspoonful of lemon juice, pepper and salt

to taste. Pick and wash the lentils, and cook them in only as much water as they will absorb. Peel, wash, and cut up the mushrooms, chop fine the onion, and fry both in the butter. Add them to the lentils now cooking; also the lemon juice and seasoning. When the lentils are quite soft, the whole should be a fairly firm pureé. Let it cool, and meanwhile make a paste of 6 oz. of Allinson fine wheatmeal and 2 oz. of butter or vege-butter and a little water. Roll the paste out thin, cut into squares of about 4 inches. Place some of the lentil mixture in each, moisten the edges, turn half over, and press the edges together. Bake for 15 minutes in a floured tin, and serve with brown sauce, vegetables, and potatoes.

LENTILS (CURRIED), AND RICE.

1 breakfastcupful each of lentils and rice, 1 lb. of fresh tomatoes or ½ a tinful of tinned ones, 1 dessertspoonful of curry, 3 eggs, well beaten, 2 oz. of butter, some breadcrumbs, and salt to taste. Roast the rice in a frying-pan in half of the butter until browned; then set it over the fire with 1-1/2 pints of water and the lentils, picked and washed. When tender set them aside to cool a little. Scald and skin the tomatoes, cut them into slices and place them in a buttered pie-dish. Smooth the curry with 1 spoonful of water; add the curry, the eggs, and salt to the cooked rice and lentils, and mix all well. Spread all over the tomatoes, scatter breadcrumbs over the top, cut up the rest of the butter in pieces and place them here and there over the breadcrumbs. Bake the savoury for ¾ of an hour to 1 hour.

LENTILS (POTTED), FOR SANDWICHES.

½ lb. of lentils, 1 English onion, ½ a cupful of tinned tomatoes, 1 blade of mace, 1 oz. of butter, pepper and salt to taste. Pick and wash the lentils, and set them over the fire to cook, only just covered with water, adding the mace, pepper, and salt. Chop fine the onion and fry it a nice brown in the butter; add the fried onions and tomatoes to the lentils, stir them sometimes to prevent burning, and let the lentils cook gently until they have become soft and make a fairly firm purée. If too dry, add a little more water as may be required. When they are done remove the mace and turn the lentils out to get cold. Then use for making sandwiches with very thin bread and butter.

MINESTRA.

1 breakfastcupful of potatoes cut into small dice, 2 breakfastcupfuls of flagolet beans, onions, carrots, and celery mixed (the latter cut up small), ¼ lb. of rice, 2 oz. of butter, 2 oz. of grated Parmesan cheese, pepper and salt to taste. Boil the vegetables in 1 quart of water until quite tender, add the rice, also pepper and salt, and cook all together gently until the rice is soft, adding more water if necessary. Before serving add the butter and cheese, stir a few minutes, and serve.

MUSHROOM CUTLETS.

¼ lb. of mushrooms, ½ teacupful of mashed potatoes, 1 teacupful of breadcrumbs, 1 small onion, 2 eggs, 2 oz. of butter, a little milk, 1 teaspoonful of finely chopped parsley, ½ teaspoonful of herbs. Peel and cut up the mushrooms, chop up the onion, and fry them in 1 oz. of butter. Mix the mushrooms and onion with the breadcrumbs, 1 egg well beaten, add also pepper and salt to taste; if necessary add a little milk to make it into a paste; shape the mixture into cutlets, dip them in the other egg well beaten, and fry them in the rest of the butter. Serve with tomato sauce.

MUSHROOM PIE.

1-1/2 lbs. of mushrooms, 1-1/2 lbs. of potatoes, 1 Spanish onion, 1 oz. of butter, pepper and salt to taste, 1 teaspoonful of mixed herbs, and 3 hard-boiled eggs. Peel and wash the mushrooms, and cut them into 2 or 4 pieces, according to their size. Peel and wash the potatoes, and cut them into pieces the size of walnuts; parboil them with 1 pint of water, and turn them into a pie-dish with the water. Chop up the onion, and cook the mushrooms and onion for 10 minutes with the butter in ½ pint of water, adding the herbs and seasoning. Mix all well in the pie-dish, quarter the eggs, and place them on the top, cover with a short crust, and bake the pie for ¾ of an hour to 1 hour.

MUSHROOM SAVOURY.

4 ounces of Allinson plain rusks 3 eggs, 1 pint of milk, 2 oz. of butter, 1 lb. of mushrooms, 1 small onion chopped fine, and pepper and salt to taste. Crush the rusks and soak in the milk; add the eggs well whipped. Peel, wash, and cut up the mushrooms, and fry them and the onion in the butter. When they have cooked in the butter for 10 minutes add them to the other ingredients, and season with pepper and salt. Pour the mixture into a greased pie-dish, and bake the savoury for 1 hour. Serve with green vegetables, potatoes, and tomato sauce.

MUSHROOM TARTLETS.

½ lb. of mushrooms, 1 oz. of butter, 1 small English onion, 1 tablespoonful of vermicelli broken up small, pepper and salt to taste. Peel and wash the mushrooms and cut them up; chop up the onions very fine, melt the butter in the frying-pan and fry the mushrooms and onion in it, adding pepper and salt to taste; a good deal of liquid will run from the mushrooms, stir into it the vermicelli, which let cook in the juice until tender; let the mixture cool, line some tartlet tins with Allinson wholemeal crust, fill with the mixture, cover with crust, and press the edges well together; bake in a moderate oven.

MUSHROOM TART AND GRAVY.

1 lb. of mushrooms, ½ lb. of Allinson fine wheatmeal, 4 oz. of butter or Allinson frying oil, pepper and salt to taste. Pick and wash the mushrooms, remove the stalks, dry them and cut them into pieces; make pastry with the meal, 3 oz. of the butter, and a little cold water; roll it out, line a large plate and heap the mushrooms upon it, dredge well with pepper and salt, and cut the rest of the butter into bits to be scattered over the mushrooms; when you line the plate, keep a little of the paste, cut this into thin strips and lay them in diamond shape across the pie; bake the pie ¾ hour in a moderate oven.

The Gravy.—The stalks of the mushrooms, 4 eschalots chopped very fine, 1 teaspoonful of Allinson cornflour, 3 bay leaves, ½ oz. of butter, pepper and salt to taste. Fry the stalks and eschalots in the butter, then gently cook them in ¾ pint of water for ½ hour, adding seasoning and the bay leaves; strain, return the sauce to the saucepan, and thicken it with the cornflour.

MUSHROOM TURNOVERS.

½ lb. of medium-sized mushrooms, 1 oz. of butter, pepper and salt to taste. For the pastry, ½ lb. of Allinson fine wheatmeal, 3 oz. of butter (or 3 tablespoonfuls of Allinson frying oil). Make the pastry of the meal, butter, and a little water; pick and wash the mushrooms, cut them up in small pieces dredge them with pepper and salt, and fry them in the butter for

5 to 10 minutes. Roll the paste out, cut it in squares of about 4 inches, and place as much mushroom on each as it will conveniently hold. Press the edges of each square together, folding them in triangular shape, and bake them in a moderate oven for an hour. Serve with brown gravy.

OATMEAL PIE-CRUST.

4 oz. each of medium oatmeal and Allinson fine wheatmeal, and 2-1/2 oz. of vege-butter or butter. Make the crust in the usual way with cold water. It will be found beautifully short, very tasty, and more digestible than white flour pastry.

ONION TART.

1 lb. of Spanish onions, 1 lb. of English onions, 4 oz. of butter, 3 eggs, ½ pint of cream, pepper and salt to taste, ½ lb. of Allinson fine wheatmeal. Slice the onions, and stew them with 1-1/2 oz. of butter without browning them. When tender let the onions cool, mix with them the eggs, well beaten, and the cream, also the seasoning. Make a paste with the meal and the rest of the butter, line with it a baking-tin, keeping back a small quantity of the paste; pour the mixture of onions, eggs, and cream into the paste-lined tin, cut the rest of the paste into thin strips, and lay these crossways over the tart, forming diamond-shaped squares; bake the tart in a moderate oven until golden brown.

ONION TURNOVER.

2 medium-sized Spanish onions, 1 oz. of butter (or Allinson frying oil), 3 eggs, pepper and salt. For the pastry, 6 oz. of Allinson fine wheatmeal, 2-1/2 oz. of butter or oil. Chop the onions fine, boil them a few minutes in a little water, and drain them; stew them in the butter

for 10 minutes, adding the seasoning beat up the eggs and mix them well with the onions over the fire, remove the mixture as it begins to set. Have ready the pastry made with the meal, butter, and a little cold water, roll it out, place the onions and eggs on it, fold the pastry over, pinching the edges over, and bake the turnover brown. Serve with gravy. This is a Turkish dish.

POTATO PIE.

Slice potatoes and onions, stew with a little water until nearly done, put into a pie-dish, flavour with herbs, pepper, and salt, add a little soaked tapioca and very little butter, cover with short wheatmeal crust, and bake 1 hour. To make a very plain pie-crust use about 2 oz. of butter or a proportionate quantity of Allinson frying oil to 1 lb. of wheatmeal. Roll or touch with the fingers as little as possible, and mix with milk instead of water. Eat this pie with green vegetables.

POTATO AND TOMATO PIE.

2 lbs. of potatoes, 2 lbs. of tomatoes, 3 hard-boiled eggs, 1 oz. of vermicelli or sago, 1 Spanish onion, 1 dessertspoonful of thyme, 1 oz. of butter, pepper and salt to taste. For the crust, ½ lb. of Allinson fine wheatmeal, 3 oz. of butter, and as much cold water as needed. Boil the potatoes in their skins, and when nearly soft drain, peel, and cut them into pieces, scald and skin the tomatoes and cut them into pieces also. Mix them with the potatoes in a pie-dish. Chop up roughly the onion, and boil in about 1 pint of water, adding the butter and the vermicelli or sago. Cook until soft. Add pepper and salt, and mix all with the potatoes and tomatoes. Sprinkle in the thyme, and mix all the ingredients well. Quarter the eggs and place the pieces on the top of the vegetables. Make the crust, cover the dish with it, and

bake the pie from ¾ of an hour to 1 hour. The crust looks better if brushed over with white of egg before baking.

POTATOES AND MUSHROOM STEW.

1-1/2 lbs. of potatoes, 1 Spanish onion, ½ lb. of mushrooms, 1 oz. of butter, pepper and salt, and 1 teaspoonful of Allinson cornflour for thickening. Peel, wash, and cut into pieces the potatoes; chop up the onion, and set both over the fire with 1 pint of water, the butter and seasoning; let cook until the potatoes are about half done. Meanwhile skin, wash, and cut into pieces the mushrooms, add them to the other ingredients, and let all stew together until tender. Thicken the liquid with the cornflour, boil up, and serve.

QUEEN'S APPLE AND ONION PIE.

3 breakfastcupfuls of Allinson breadcrumbs, 3 eggs, 1-1/2 lbs. of apples, 2 lbs. of Spanish onions, 2 oz. of butter, ½ teaspoonful of spice, pepper and salt to taste, and a little hot milk; cut into slices the onions and apples, stew them gently (without adding-water) with 1 oz. of the butter, the spice and seasoning until quite tender. Mix the breadcrumbs with the eggs, well beaten, and enough hot milk to smooth the breadcrumbs; butter a pie-dish with ½ oz. of butter, place a layer of breadcrumbs in your dish, a layer of apple and onion, repeat this until your dish is full, finishing with breadcrumbs. Place the rest of the butter on the top in little bits, and bake the pie for 1 hour. Serve with brown gravy.

QUEEN'S ONION PIE.

3 lbs of Spanish onions, 3 breakfastcupfuls of Allinson breadcrumbs, 3 eggs, 3 oz. of butter, 1 teaspoonful of mixed herbs, 1 tablespoonful of finely chopped parsley, pepper and salt to

taste, and a little hot milk. Stew the onions in 2 oz. of butter, adding the herbs and seasoning. Prepare the breadcrumbs in the same way as for "Queen's Onion and Apple Pie," place the onions and breadcrumbs in layers as in the previous recipe, and bake 1 hour.

QUEEN'S TOMATO PIE.

8 breakfastcupfuls of Allinson breadcrumbs, 3 eggs, 2 lbs. of tomatoes, 2 finely chopped onions, ½ oz. of butter, pepper and salt to taste, a little boiling milk; 1 dessertspoonful of finely chopped parsley. Cut the tomatoes into slices, and stew them gently with 1 oz. of the butter, the onions and seasoning for 10 minutes, then add the parsley. Soak the breadcrumbs with enough hot milk to just moisten them through, add the eggs beaten up. Grease a pie-dish, place in it first a layer of breadcrumbs, then one of tomatoes and so on until full, finishing with breadcrumbs. Put the rest of the butter in little bits on the top of the pie, and bake it until lightly brown.

SAVOURY CUSTARD.

1 quart of milk; 6 eggs, 6 oz. of grated cheese, Parmesan is the best, but any kind of cooking cheese can be used; ½ a saltspoonful of nutmeg, pepper and salt to taste. Heat the milk; meanwhile whip the eggs well, and mix the cheese and seasoning with them. Mix well with the hot milk, pour the mixture into a buttered pie-dish, and bake in a moderately hot oven until set. Serve with green vegetables and potatoes.

SAVOURY CUSTARD (Another way).

1 quart of milk, 6 eggs, pepper and salt to taste, 1 tablespoonful each of finely chopped parsley and spring onion. Proceed as above;

mix the herbs and onion with the custard, and bake until set.

SAVOURY FRITTERS (1).

1 teacupful of mashed potatoes, ½ lb. of breadcrumbs, 1 large English onion, 2 eggs, 1 oz. of butter, 1 teaspoonful of powdered sage, ½ saltspoonful of nutmeg, pepper and salt to taste. Chop the onion up fine and fry it brown in the butter. Whip up the eggs and mix both ingredients with the breadcrumbs; add the mashed potatoes, herbs, and seasoning, and mix all well together. Form into fritters, dredge with flour, and fry them a nice brown. Serve with vegetables, potatoes, and sauce.

SAVOURY FRITTERS (2).

12 oz. of onions, 6 oz. of breadcrumbs, 1 teaspoonful of dried sage, 2 eggs, 1-1/2 oz. of butter, pepper and salt to taste. Chop the onions up small and fry them in the butter, or oil a nice brown, then add the sage to them. Mix a third of the onions with the breadcrumbs, add the eggs well beaten, pepper and salt; mix all well, form into fritters, and fry in butter or oil. The remainder of the onions place round the fritters on the dish. Serve with apple sauce.

SAVOURY PICKLED WALNUT.

½ lb. of Allinson bread, 1 pint of milk, 3 eggs, 4 pickled walnuts and the vinegar to taste, 1 tablespoonful of finely chopped parsley, 1 teaspoonful of powdered mixed herbs, 1 grated English onion, 2 oz. of butter, pepper and salt to taste. Soak the bread in the milk, add the parsley, herbs, onion, eggs and seasoning. Mash up the pickled walnuts, dissolve part of the butter on the stove and add both to the other ingredients; mix all well. Butter a pie-dish with the rest of the butter, pour in the mixture, and bake.

SAVOURY PIE.

6 oz. of haricot beans, ½ lb. of onions, 1 lb. of tomatoes, ½ lb. of parboiled potatoes, 2 hard-boiled eggs, 1 teaspoonful of herbs, 4 oz. of butter, ½ lb. of fine wheatmeal, pepper and salt to taste. Have the beans boiled the previous day, place them in a pie-dish, chop up the onions and boil them in a little water until soft, cut the potatoes in small dice, slice the tomatoes, cut up the eggs, and mix all the ingredients thoroughly in the pie dish, adding the herbs, 1 oz. of butter, and seasoning. Pour over the mixture 1 pint of water, and let it cook for 1 hour in the oven. Make a paste of the wheatmeal, the rest of the butter and a little cold water, cover the vegetables with it, and bake the pie 1 hour in a moderate oven.

SAVOURY TARTLETS.

4 eggs, 4 oz. grated cheese, 1 oz. of butter, 1 teaspoonful of mustard, 1 gill of cream, pepper and salt to taste. For the crust 6 oz. of Allinson fine wheatmeal, and 2 oz. of butter. Whip up the eggs and add to each egg 1 dessertspoonful of water. Dissolve the mustard in a little water; mix this, the cheese and seasoning with the eggs. Heat the butter in a frying-pan, and when boiling stir in the eggs and cheese mixture, stirring it with a knife over the fire until set. Turn the mixture into a bowl to cool. Meanwhile have ready the paste for the pastry. Rub the butter into the flour, add enough water to make it hold together, mixing the paste with a knife. Roll it out thin, line small patty pans, fill with the egg and cheese mixture. Moisten the edges of the paste in the patty pans, cover with paste, and press the edges together. Bake the little tartlets in a

moderately hot oven until done; they will take from 15 to 20 minutes.

SPAGHETTI AUX TOMATOES.

1 lb. of spaghetti, the strained juice of one tin of tomatoes, 1 oz. of butter, pepper and salt. Mix the tomato juice with 1 pint of water and let the liquid come to the boil, throw in the spaghetti, taking care to keep the contents of the saucepan boiling fast; add the butter and seasoning, and cook until tender; time from 15 to 20 minutes. Serve very hot with grated cheese.

SPANISH ONIONS (Stewed).

Cut up lengthways as many onions as may be required, according to number in family. Set them over a fire in a saucepan with a piece of butter the size of a walnut, and 1 teacupful of water; let them stew gently for 1 1/2 hours, when there will be a lot of juice boiled out of the onions. Chop fine a handful of parsley, thicken the liquid on the onions with some Allinson fine wheatmeal, add pepper and salt; let the onions simmer a few minutes longer, then mix the parsley with them, and serve at once with squares of toast. This is a very nice dish for the evening meal.

SPANISH ONIONS AND CHEESE.

This is a very savoury dish and suitable for an evening meal. 1 lb. of Spanish onions, 4 oz. of cheese, a few breadcrumbs, pepper and salt to taste, and 1 oz. of butter. Peel and slice the onions thinly and grate the cheese. Arrange the onions in a pie-dish in layers, sprinkling cheese and a little pepper and salt between each layer. Finish with the cheese, scatter breadcrumbs on the top, cut up the butter into bits and scatter it over the breadcrumbs. Pour a small teacupful of water into the pie-dish, and bake about 2 hours. This is nice eaten cold as well as hot.

SPANISH ONIONS AND WHITE SAUCE.

Choose as many onions of equal size as are required and boil them whole in plenty of water until tender; the time necessary being about 2 to 2-1/2 hours. Then drain them, keeping the water they were boiled in as stock for soup or stew. Make the sauce as follows: ½ pint of milk, 1 oz. of butter, 1 heaped teaspoonful of cornflour, pepper and salt to taste. Boil the milk with the butter and seasoning, and thicken it with the cornflour. Boil the sauce up again and pour it over the onions, which should be ready on a hot dish on slices of toast.

SPANISH STEW.

2 lbs. of potatoes, 1 lb. of Spanish onions, 1 lb. of tomatoes, 2 oz. of vermicelli, ½ pint of milk, 1 oz. of butter, pepper and salt. Cut up into dice the potatoes and onions, and stew them with the butter and very little water; when they are tender, add the tomatoes cut in slices, and cook the vegetables 10 minutes longer. Add seasoning, the milk and vermicelli, and a little more water if necessary; let the whole simmer for another 10 minutes, and serve.

SPINACH DUMPLINGS.

2 lbs. of spinach, 3 eggs, 1 oz. of butter, 2 finely chopped onions, juice of ½ a lemon, pepper and salt, and some Allinson fine wheatmeal. Pick and wash the spinach, boil it with the onions without water until quite tender; drain it dry, chop the spinach fine, and mix it with the eggs well beaten, the lemon juice, butter, and seasoning. Add as much of

the meal as necessary to make the mixture into a soft paste. Form into balls, flour them, drop them into boiling water, and boil them 5 to 10 minutes; serve with potatoes and gravy.

STEWED MUSHROOMS.

1 lb. of mushrooms, 1 small English onion, 1 oz. of butter, 1 dessertspoonful of Allinson cornflour, ½ pint of milk, ½ pint of water, pepper and salt to taste. Peel, wash, and dry the mushrooms—if big, quarter them—chop fine the onion, and fry both in the butter for 10 minutes. Add the water, milk, and seasoning, and let it all simmer for 20 minutes; thicken with the cornflour, boil up and serve with curried or plain boiled rice.

STUFFED SPANISH ONIONS WITH BROWN SAUCE.

4 good-sized Spanish onions, 1 breakfastcupful of Allinson breadcrumbs, an egg, 1 teaspoonful of powdered dry sage, or a dessertspoonful of minced fresh sage, pepper and salt to taste, and 2 oz. of butter. Boil the onions for 20 minutes and drain them. Cut a piece off the top of each onion and scoop out enough inside to leave at least 1 inch thick of the outer part. Chop up finely the part removed, mix it with the breadcrumbs, the sage, pepper, and salt. Beat up the egg, melt 1 oz. of the butter, and mix with the breadcrumbs, and stuff the onions with the mixture. Replace the slices cut off the tops of the onions, and tie them on with white cotton. Place the onions in a pie-dish or deep tin, put the rest of the butter on the top of the onions, cover them up, and bake them until quite tender. Have ready the brown sauce, remove the threads of cotton, and pour the sauce over the cooked onions.

SWEET CORN FRITTERS.

½ tin of sweet corn, 2 eggs, ½ pint of milk, ½ oz. of Allinson fine wheatmeal, pepper, and salt, ½ saltspoonful of nutmeg, and some oil or butter. Make a batter of the meal, milk, and the eggs well beaten, adding the seasoning and the sweet corn. Have some oil (vege-butter) boiling in the frying-pan, drop spoonfuls of the batter into the boiling fat, and fry the fritters a golden brown. Serve with slices of lemon or tomato sauce.

TOMATO PIE.

1-1/2 lbs. of tomatoes, ½ lb. of onions, 1 oz. of butter, 2 oz. of vermicelli, 2 hard-boiled eggs. For the crust, 8 oz. of Allinson fine wheatmeal, 3 oz. of butter. Cut up the potatoes and onions into dice, and parboil them in 1 pint of water, adding the butter and seasoning. Turn them into a pie-dish, add the tomatoes and eggs cut in slices, mix all the ingredients, and add the vermicelli broken up small. Make a paste with the meal, butter, and a little cold water, cover the pie with the crust, and bake for 1 hour.

TOMATO TORTILLA.

1 lb. of tomatoes, 1 oz. of butter, 4 eggs, pepper and salt to taste. Scald, skin, and slice the tomatoes. Melt the butter in a frying-pan. Add it to the tomatoes with seasoning, and stew in the butter until quite tender and until a good deal of the liquid has steamed away. Whip the eggs and stir them into the cooked tomatoes; keep stirring until the mixture has thickened. Serve on hot buttered toast. This mixture can also be used cold for sandwiches.

TOMATOES À LA PARMESAN.

4 large tomatoes, 1 oz. of butter, 3 oz. of Parmesan cheese, ¾ pint of milk, 1 dessertspoonful of Allinson fine wheatmeal,

pepper and salt to taste. Bake the tomatoes in a tin with the butter and a dredging of pepper and salt. Make a sauce with the milk, meal, and cheese, seasoning it with a little cayenne pepper if handy. When the tomatoes are baked, place them on hot buttered toast, pour the sauce over, and serve hot.

TOMATOES AND ONION PIE.

Cut tomatoes and Spanish onions in slices, put into a pie-dish in alternate layers, add a little soaked tapioca, pepper and salt, and a little butter to taste. Put in sufficient water to make gravy, cover with wholemeal crust, bake 1-1/2 hours; eat with baked potatoes and bread.

TOMATOES AU GRATIN.

8 medium-sized tomatoes, 1 breakfastcupful of breadcrumbs, 1 teaspoonful each of finely chopped parsley, mint, and eschalot, 1 egg, pepper and salt, 1 oz. of butter. Make a stuffing of the breadcrumbs, parsley, mint, and eschalots, adding the egg well beaten, and seasoning. Make a small opening in the tomato and take out the seeds with a teaspoon; fill the tomatoes with the stuffing, put them into a tin, place a bit of butter on each, pour ½ a teacupful of water in the tin, and bake the tomatoes 15 minutes.

VEGETABLE BALLS.

These are an excellent addition to stews. Boil till soft, and mash up together equal quantities of potatoes, turnips, carrots, lentils, vegetable marrow, and haricot beans, and season nicely with pepper, salt, nutmeg, and mixed herbs. Bind with beaten eggs, dip in frying batter, and fry the balls in vege-butter or oil till golden brown.

VEGETABLE MOULD.

2 breakfastcupfuls of mashed potatoes, 2 ditto of parboiled finely cut turnips, carrots, celery, onion, and green peas all mixed, 2 eggs, 1 teaspoonful of mixed herbs, pepper and salt to taste. Beat the eggs up and mix all the ingredients well together; butter a mould. Fill in the mixture, cover with the lid or tie a cloth over it, and steam for 2 hours. Turn out, and serve with brown sauce.

VEGETABLE PIE (1).

½ lb. each of tomatoes, turnips, carrots, potatoes, 1 tablespoonful of sago, 1 teaspoonful of mixed herbs, 3 hard-boiled eggs, 2 oz. of butter, and pepper and salt to taste. Prepare the vegetables, scald and skin the tomatoes, cut them in pieces not bigger than a walnut, stew them in the butter and 1 pint of water until nearly tender, add the pepper and salt and the mixed herbs. When cooked, pour the vegetables into a pie-dish, sprinkle in the sago, add water to make gravy if necessary. Cut the hard-boiled eggs in quarters and place them on the top of the vegetables, cover with a crust, and bake until it is brown.

VEGETABLE PIE (2).

½ lb. each of carrots, turnips, onions, potatoes, 1 small cauliflower, 2 good sized tomatoes or a cupful of tinned ones, 2 hard-boiled eggs, 1 teaspoonful of mixed herbs, 1 oz. of butter, 1 dessertspoonful of sago, pepper and salt to taste. Wash and prepare the vegetables, cut them into pieces the size of nuts; if fresh tomatoes are used, scald and skin them. Let all the vegetables stew gently with the butter and 1 pint of water until they are nearly tender; add the herbs, and seasoning; pour the whole into a pie-dish, sprinkling the sago between the vegetables; add water if more is required for the pie to have sufficient gravy; cut up the eggs in quarters, place the pieces on the top of the vegetables, and cover all with a crust. These vegetable pies can be varied according to the vegetables in season; cooked haricot or kidney beans, lentils, green peas, French beans may be used, and vermicelli or tapioca substituted for the sago.

VEGETABLE STEW.

Fry 2 Spanish onions in 2 oz. of butter, then add 3 turnips, 2 carrots, a little white celery, and 1 pint of water. Allow all to stew for 2 hours, then mix a tablespoonful of Allinson fine wheatmeal with ½ pint of milk. Add to the stew, and serve.

YORKSHIRE PUDDING.

4 eggs, ½ lb. of Allinson fine wheatmeal, 1 pint of milk, pepper and salt to taste, 1 oz. of butter. Thoroughly beat the eggs, make a batter of them with the flour and milk, and season it. Well butter a shallow tin, pour in the batter, and cut the rest of the butter in bits. Scatter them over the batter, and bake it ¾ hour. Serve with vegetables, potatoes, and sauce. To use half each of Allinson breakfast oats and wheatmeal will be found very tasty.

NUTROAST.

1 lb. breadcrumbs, 6 oz. ground cob nuts, 2 oz. butter (oiled), 4 eggs; 1 small onion chopped very fine, 1 good pinch of mixed herbs, pepper and salt to taste, and enough milk just to smoothly moisten the mixture. Mix all the ingredients thoroughly, turn into a buttered bread tin and steam 2-1/2-3 hours; turn out and serve with brown sauce.

MACARONI

Macaroni is one of the most nutritious farinaceous foods. It is made from Italian wheat, which contains more flesh-forming matter than butcher's meat. In the manufacture of macaroni some of the bran is removed from the flour, but the meal left is still very rich in flesh-forming matter. As the coarser particles of the bran have been taken away, macaroni is slightly constipating, and must therefore always be eaten with green vegetables, onions, or fruit. Macaroni should always be boiled before being made into various dishes. It may be cooked in plain water, or in milk and water; a little salt may be added by those who use it, and care should be taken to use just enough water to cook it in, so that when the macaroni is done, little or no fluid may be left, but if any does remain it should be saved for sauce, stock for soup, &c., as it contains valuable nutritive material. Macaroni takes from 20 minutes to 1 hour to cook, according to the kind used. That which is slightly yellow is to be preferred to the white, as the latter is usually poorer than the former in mineral salts and flesh-forming substances. From 2 to 4 oz. may be regarded as the amount to be allowed at a meal for grown-up persons.

A very simple nourishing and satisfying meal can be made from macaroni plainly boiled; it may be eaten with any kind of vegetables, or baked potatoes, or fried onions, and if desired, with grated cheese, onion, caper, or parsley sauce.

MACARONI (Italian).

½ lb. of spaghetti or vermicelli, 2 oz. of butter, 2 eggs, 3 oz. of grated cheese, 1 tablespoonful of finely chopped parsley, pepper and salt to taste. Boil the macaroni till tender in 2 pints of water, to which the butter has been added. When soft add seasoning, the cheese, and the parsley. Beat the eggs well in the dish in which the macaroni is to be served, pour over the mixture of macaroni and other ingredients, mix all well with the eggs, and serve. If neither spaghetti nor vermicelli are handy, use Naples macaroni.

MACARONI CHEESE.

½ lb. of macaroni, 8 oz. of grated cheese, some breadcrumbs, pepper and salt to taste, and 1 oz. of butter. Boil the macaroni in slightly salted water until soft. Then place a layer of it in a pie-dish, sprinkle some of the grated cheese over it, dust with pepper, and repeat the layers of macaroni and cheese, finishing with a sprinkling of cheese, and the breadcrumbs. Cut the butter in pieces, and place them here and there on the top. Bake it in a moderately hot oven until brown. Eat with vegetables and tomato sauce. For those who have a weak digestion plain boiled macaroni with grated cheese added at table is better and lighter. Macaroni requires from 25 minutes to ½ an hour cooking. The Genoa macaroni takes longer, the thin spaghetti kind is done in from 15 to 20 minutes, and vermicelli and Italian paste are done in a few minutes. Macaroni should be thrown into boiling water and be kept boiling, as the pipes or pieces otherwise stick together. The Italian paste is mostly used as an addition in clear soup.

MACARONI CREAM.

6 oz. of macaroni, 3 oz. of cheese, ½ oz. of butter, ¾ pint of milk, 1 teaspoonful of Allinson cornflour, pepper and salt to taste. Boil the macaroni until tender in only as much water as it will absorb. Make a sauce of the milk, cornflour, and cheese (you can use Parmesan, Gruyère, or Canadian cheese). Place the

macaroni in a pie-dish, pour the sauce over it, grate some more cheese over the top, and let the macaroni brown in the oven.

MACARONI SAVOURY.

4 oz. of boiled macaroni, 4 oz. of Allinson fine wheatmeal, 3 eggs, ¾ pint of milk, 1 finely chopped onion, the grated rind of 1 lemon, 2 oz. of grated cheese, 1 tablespoonful of finely chopped parsley, 1 oz. of butter, ½ a saltspoonful of grated nutmeg, pepper and salt to taste. Cut the macaroni in small pieces. Make a batter of the milk, eggs, and meal, mix into it all the other ingredients, pour it into a buttered pie-dish, cut up the butter in pieces and spread them on the top. Bake the savoury for 1 to 1-1/2 hours.

RICE

In many households it seems a difficulty to get rice cooked properly, that is having all the grains separate. Very often it comes to table in a soft, pulpy mass, which is certainly not appetising. To cook it in a large saucepanful of water which is then drained away is very wasteful, for a great deal of the goodness of the rice is thrown away. The following recipe will be found thoroughly reliable and satisfactory.

RICE, HOW TO COOK.

1 lb. of good rice, 1 quart of water, 1 oz. of butter, salt to taste. Wash the rice and set it over the fire with 1 quart of cold water, the butter and salt. Let it come to the boil gently, stirring it a little to prevent the rice from sticking to the saucepan. When the rice boils, set it on the side and let it just simmer. It will be sufficiently cooked in 15 to 20 minutes and

each grain will be separate. Rice should not be cooked too soft, only just cooked through.

CURRIED RICE.

1 lb. of Patna rice, 1 quart of cold water, 1 dessertspoonful of curry, 1 oz. of butter, and salt to taste. Wash the rice, mix the curry with the proper quantity of water, and set the rice over the fire with it, adding the butter and seasoning. Let the rice come to the boil slowly, and stir it a few times to prevent it sticking to the saucepan. When the rice boils, cover it with a piece of buttered paper, and let it cook very gently, not stirring it again. When all the water is absorbed, serve the rice. Do not allow it to get very soft; the rice will take from 15 to 20 minutes' cooking only.

CURRIED RICE AND TOMATOES.

½ lb. of Patna rice, 1 dessertspoonful of curry powder, salt to taste, and 1 oz. of butter. Wash the rice; mix 1 pint of cold water with the curry powder, put this over the fire with the rice, butter, and salt. Cover the rice with a piece of buttered paper and let it simmer gently until the water is absorbed. This will take about 20 minutes. Rice cooked this way will have all the grains separate. For the tomatoes proceed as follows: 1 lb. of tomatoes and a little butter, pepper and salt. Wash the tomatoes and place them in a flat tin with a few spoonfuls of water; dust them with pepper and salt, and place little bits of butter on each tomato. Bake them from 15 to 20 minutes, according to the size of the tomatoes and the heat of the oven. Place the rice in the centre of a hot flat dish, put the tomatoes round it, pour the liquid over the rice, and serve.

PORTUGUESE RICE.

1 teacupful of rice, 3 medium-sized onions, 3 tomatoes, 2 oz. of grated cheese, ½ teaspoonful of herbs, 1 oz. of butter, pepper and salt to taste. Peel and slice the onions and tomatoes and fry them in the butter for 15 minutes; place the rice over the fire with 1 pint of water; add the onions, tomatoes, herbs, and seasoning, and let all cook until the rice is quite soft; serve in a vegetable dish with the grated cheese sprinkled over.

RICE AND LENTILS.

Boil the rice as above; stew Egyptian lentils with chopped onions, pepper, salt, and a little butter, until well done. Put the rice on a dish, pour over the stewed onions and lentils, serve, and eat with green vegetables.

RICE AND ONIONS.

Boil whole onions in water until done quite through, remove them from the water, and put in it washed rice with a little pepper, salt, and butter. When done, serve with the onions and eat with a green vegetable.

SAVOURY RICE (Italian).

1 breakfastcupful of rice, 4 tablespoonfuls of grated cheese (Parmesan or other cheese), 1 oz. of butter, a pinch of saffron, pepper and salt to taste. Boil the rice with water as above, then add the cheese, butter, saffron, and seasoning; mix all well, and serve.

SAVOURY RICE CROQUETTES.

½ lb. of Patna rice, 1-1/2 pints of milk, 1 lb. of Spanish onions, 1 oz. of butter, 2 eggs, 1 teacupful of raspings, Allinson's oil for frying. Boil the rice in the milk until soft, and turn it out to get quite cold. Meanwhile chop the onions up fine and fry them brown in the butter. Form the cold rice into balls, and with the thumb of the right hand hollow them sufficiently to admit of their receiving a stuffing of fried onions, close them again carefully, dip them in the eggs beaten up and then in the raspings, and fry them in boiling oil a light brown. Serve with gravy. There are various stuffings which can be used instead of the onions—fried mushrooms chopped up, some olives chopped fine and mixed with hard-boiled yolks of eggs, &c.

SPANISH RICE.

6 onions, 6 tomatoes, 1-1/2 pints of vegetable stock, herbs and seasoning, 1-1/2 cupfuls of rice, butter. Fry the onions and tomatoes in butter until well browned, then place them with the seasoning into the cold stock, and add the rice. When all have boiled slowly for 20 minutes, the rice should have absorbed the stock. Serve with cheese grated over.

OMELETS

CHEESE OMELET.

4 slices of Allinson bread toasted, or Allinson rusks, 3 eggs, ¼ lb. of grated cheese, 1 saltspoonful of nutmeg, 1 pint of milk, 2 oz. of butter, pepper and salt to taste. Beat up the eggs, and mix them with the milk; crush the toast or rusks with your hands, and soak them in the egg and milk. Add the cheese, nutmeg, and seasoning. Dissolve half of the butter and mix it with the other ingredients. Butter a pie-dish, pour in the mixture, cut the rest of the butter in little pieces, and scatter them over the top. Bake the savoury for 1 hour or a little longer until well set. Serve hot or cold.

FRENCH BEAN OMELET.

3 tablespoonfuls of cut boiled French beans, 4 eggs, 1 dessertspoonful of Allinson fine wheatmeal, ½ a teacupful of milk, 2 tablespoonfuls of grated cheese (Gruyère or Parmesan), pepper and salt to taste, some vege-butter or oil for frying. Smooth the meal with the milk, beat up the eggs and add them, the cheese and seasoning to the meal and milk; mix thoroughly with the beans, and fry the omelet in boiling butter or Allinson frying oil.

FRENCH OMELET WITH CHEESE.

3 eggs, 1 oz. of grated cheese, 3 dessertspoonfuls of water, pepper and salt to taste, and 1 oz. of butter. Beat the yolks of the eggs, add to them the water and seasoning; whip the whites of the eggs to a stiff froth, and mix it lightly with the yolks. Meanwhile have the butter boiling hot in an omelet pan, pour the mixture into it, and let it fry over a gentle fire. Pass a heated salamander or coal-shovel over the top of the omelet. When it has risen, scatter the cheese over it; let the omelet cook a little longer, fold over when the top is still creamy, and serve immediately.

GARDENER'S OMELET.

1 breakfastcupful of cold boiled vegetables, minced fine (green peas, carrots, turnips, potatoes, &c.), 4 eggs, 1 tablespoonful of Allinson fine wheatmeal, ½ a gill of milk, pepper and salt, and a little nutmeg to taste, 1 oz. of butter. Beat the eggs and milk well together, rub the meal smooth with it, add the vegetables and seasoning, and fry as an omelet. Serve with sauce.

OMELET HERB.

4 slices of Allinson bread, 1 pint of milk, 1 finely chopped English onion, 1 good

tablespoonful of finely chopped parsley, 1 teaspoonful of dried mixed herbs, 3 eggs, 2 oz. of butter, pepper and salt to taste. Soak the bread, fry the onion in 1-1/2 oz. of butter, and mix it with the soaked bread. Add the herbs, parsley, and seasoning, and mix all well. Butter a pie-dish with the rest of the butter, pour the mixture into it, and bake.

OMELET LENTIL.

It you have any cold boiled lentils, for instance, some sandwich mixture you wish to use up, proceed as follows: To 1 teacupful of boiled lentils take 3 well-beaten eggs, and pepper and salt to taste. Add 1 dessertspoonful of water to each egg, and mix the lentils and eggs smooth. Fry the mixture as an omelet in boiling butter.

OMELET MACARONI.

3 oz. of boiled cold macaroni, 3 eggs, 1 dessertspoonful of finely chopped parsley, 1-1/2 oz. of grated cheese, ½ a saltspoonful of nutmeg, pepper and salt to taste, 1-1/2 oz. of butter. Cut the macaroni into little pieces; beat the eggs well, and mix them with the macaroni. Add the seasoning, parsley, cheese, and nutmeg; mix all well, and fry the omelet with the butter in a large frying-pan.

OMELET ONION.

4 medium-sized English onions, 1-1/2 oz. of butter, 2 oz. of Allinson breadcrumbs, 4 eggs, 4 tablespoonfuls of milk, pepper and salt to taste. Peel and slice the onions, bake them in a pie-dish with the butter and seasoning, until quite soft. Whip the eggs up, mix them with the milk, breadcrumbs, and the baked onions. Put the mixture into a greased pie-dish, and bake in a moderately hot oven. Serve with tomato sauce.

OMELET SAVOURY.

Soak Allinson wholemeal bread in cold milk and water until soft, then rub smooth, grate 1 onion, beat up 1 egg, and add a few flavouring herbs, and pepper and salt to taste. Mix the whole together, put in a pie-dish, place a few small pieces of butter on the top, and bake about ½ hour, or until done. Eat with vegetables and potatoes.

OMELET SOUFFLÉ.

4 eggs, 3 oz. of sifted castor sugar, the grated rind of ½ a lemon, 1 oz. of butter. Beat the yolks of the eggs for 10 minutes with the sugar and lemon rind. Whip the whites of the eggs to a very stiff froth, mix it with the other ingredients, pour the mixture into a well-buttered pie-dish or cake tin, and bake the Soufflé in a moderately hot oven from 10 to 15 minutes. Serve immediately.

OMELET SOUFFLÉ (SWEET).

6 eggs, 3 oz. of powdered sugar, 1 oz. of butter, 1 dessertspoonful of potato flour, and 1 dessertspoonful of orangeflower water. Put the yolks of the eggs into a large basin, add the sugar, potato flour, and orange water, and beat all well with a wooden spoon for 10 minutes; beat the whites of the eggs to a stiff froth, and mix them lightly with the other ingredients. Meanwhile beat the butter in the omelet pan; when boiling pour the mixture into it, and fry the omelet over a gentle fire. When it begins to set round the sides shake it very gently from side to side, and turn the omelet neatly out on a buttered dish. Set it in the oven for about 10 minutes, and serve immediately with a little castor sugar sifted over it.

OMELET TOMATO (1).

This is made in almost the same way as the savoury omelet, but without the addition of flavouring herbs. 2 average-sized tomatoes are cut up fine, and mixed with the ingredients given above. When tinned tomatoes are used the juice may be made hot and the bread soaked in it instead of in milk and water.

OMELET TOMATO (2).

1 lb. of tomatoes, ½ lb. of breadcrumbs, 1 large Spanish onion, 3 eggs, 2 oz. of butter, pepper and salt to taste. Stew the finely chopped onions in the butter for 20 minutes in a covered-up saucepan, add pepper and salt, cut the tomatoes up, add these to the other ingredients. Let all simmer for 20 minutes; pour the mixture over the breadcrumbs, add the eggs well beaten, mix all up thoroughly, and turn the mixture into one or more well-buttered shallow tins. Bake the omelet in a quick oven for 10 to 15 minutes.

OMELET TRAPPIST.

4 oz. of fine breadcrumbs, 2 eggs, 1-1/2 oz. of butter, ½ teaspoonful of powdered herbs, pepper and salt to taste, ½ gill of boiling milk. Moisten the breadcrumbs with the milk, add the eggs well beaten, the herbs and seasoning. Mix all well and smoothly. Melt the butter in the frying-pan, spread the mixture in it, and fry the omelet a golden brown both sides.

SWEET OMELET (1).

3 eggs, 2 oz. of butter, sugar to taste, 1 lemon, and ½ a teacupful of new milk. Whip the yolks of the eggs well, adding the grated rind of the lemon, half the butter melted, the milk, and sugar. Just before frying the omelet, add the lemon juice and the whites of the eggs whipped to a stiff froth. Make the rest of the butter boiling hot in an oval omelet pan, the

size of the dish on which it is to be served, and fry till lightly browned. Sift sugar over it, and serve immediately.

SWEET OMELET (2).

½ pint of new milk, 4 eggs, cinnamon and sugar to taste, 1 oz. of butter, and 1 teaspoonful of Allinson fine wheatmeal. Smooth the wheatmeal with the milk, and mix with the other ingredients. Make the butter boiling hot in a frying-pan, and fry the omelet till lightly browned. Serve immediately with sugar sifted over it.

SWEET OMELET (3).

5 eggs, 1 tablespoonful of castor sugar, 2 tablespoonfuls of water, 2 oz. of butter, some raspberry and currant jam. Melt the butter in an omelet pan, beat the eggs well, stir in the sugar, and pour the mixture into the hot butter. Fry a pale golden colour, and turn it on to a hot dish. Spread some jam on the omelet, double it, and serve at once. The inside of the omelet should remain creamy.

VEGETABLES

GREEN VEGETABLES (General Remarks).

I have not given recipes for the cooking of plain greens, as they are prepared very much alike everywhere in England. There are a number of recipes in this book giving savoury ways of preparing them, and I will now make a few remarks on the cooking of plain vegetables. The English way of boiling them is not at all a good one, as most of the soluble vegetable salts, which are so important to our system, are lost through it. Green vegetables are generally boiled in a great deal of salt water; this is drained off when they are tender, and the vegetables then served. A much better way for all vegetables is to cook them in a very small quantity of water, and adding a small piece of butter (1 oz. to 2 lb. of greens) and a little salt. When the greens are tender, any water which is not absorbed should be thickened with a little Allinson fine wheatmeal and eaten with the vegetables. A great number of them, such as *Cabbages, Savoys, Brussel sprouts, Scotch kail, turnip-tops, &c., &c.*, can be prepared this way.

In the case of vegetables like *asparagus, cauliflower, sea kale, parsnips, artichokes, carrots* or *celery*, which cannot always be stewed in a little water, this should be saved as stock for soups or sauces. Most of these vegetables are very nice with a white sauce; carrots are particularly pleasant with parsley sauce.

Spinach is a vegetable which English cooks rarely prepare nicely; the Continental way of preparing it is as follows: The spinach is cooked without water, with a little salt; when quite tender it is strained, turned on to a board, and chopped very finely; then it is returned to the saucepan with a piece of butter, a little nutmeg, or a few very finely chopped eschalots and some of the juice previously strained. When the spinach is cooking a little Allinson fine wheatmeal, smoothed in 1 or 2 tablespoonfuls of milk, is added to bind the spinach with the juice; cook it a few minutes longer, and serve it with slices of hard-boiled egg on the top. *Potatoes* also require a good deal of care. When peeled, potatoes are plainly boiled, they should be placed over the fire after the water has been strained; the potatoes should be lightly shaken to allow the moisture to steam out. This makes them mealy and more palatable. Potatoes which have been baked in their skins should be pricked when tender, or the skins be cracked in some way, otherwise they very soon become sodden. A very palatable way of serving potatoes, is to peel them and bake them in a tin with a little oil or butter, or vege-butter; they should be turned occasionally, in order that they should brown evenly. This is not a very hygienic way of preparing potatoes. From a health point of view they are best baked in their skins, or steamed with or without the skins. A good many vegetables may be steamed with advantage; for instance, *cabbage, sprouts, turnips, parsnips, swedes, Scotch kail, &c.* Any way of preparing greens is better than boiling them in a large saucepanful of water and throwing this away. I may just mention that Scotch kail, after being boiled in a little water, should be treated exactly as spinach, and is most delicious in that way; an onion cooked with it greatly improves the flavour.

ARTICHOKES À LA SAUCE BLANCHE.

2 lbs. of artichokes, 1 oz. of Allinson fine wheatmeal, ¾ pint of milk, 1 egg, juice of ½ a lemon, pepper and salt to taste. Peel the artichokes, and boil them in water until tender; cut them into slices ½ an inch thick and place them on a dish. Make a sauce of the milk and meal with seasoning; when the sauce has thickened, remove it from the fire, beat up the egg with the lemon juice and add both to the sauce, pour it over the artichokes, and serve.

ARTICHOKES À LA PARMESAN.

2 lbs. of artichokes, ¾ pint of milk, 1 tablespoonful of Allinson fine wheatmeal, 1 egg, juice of ½ a lemon, 2 oz. of grated Parmesan or any other cooking cheese. Proceed as in the recipe for "Celery à la Parmesan," add the cheese to the sauce, and serve the same with sauce as above.

ASPARAGUS (BOILED).

Scrape the white parts of the stalks quite clean, and put them into cold water as they are done. Tie them up into bundles, and cut them all the same length. Now put them into a saucepan, cover with boiling water, add a little salt, and boil gently and steadily for 20 to 30 minutes. Take them out of the water as soon as they are tender, and dish on to rounds of toast with the points to the middle. Serve with them rich melted butter in a tureen.

CABBAGE.

Remove the outer coarse leaves, cut the cabbage in four pieces lengthways, and well wash the pieces in salt water. The salt is added because it kills any insects which may be present. Wash the cabbage as often as is necessary in pure water after this to clean it and remove the salt, and then shred it up fine. Set it over the fire with ½ pint of water, 1 oz. of butter, a dash of pepper, and a very little salt. Let it cook very gently for 2 hours; when it is quite tender, the liquid can be thickened with a little fine wheatmeal; smooth this with a little milk, or water if milk is not handy; boil it up, and serve.

CARROTS WITH PARSLEY SAUCE.

Scrub and wash as many carrots as are required. Cook them in a little water or steam them until quite tender, then slice them and place them in a saucepan. Make a white sauce as directed in the recipe for "Onions and white sauce," and stir into it a handful of finely-chopped parsley. Pour the sauce over the carrots, and let them simmer for ten minutes. Serve very hot with baked potatoes.

CAULIFLOWER WITH WHITE SAUCE.

Trim the cauliflower, cutting away only the bad and bruised leaves and the coarse part of the stalk. Put it into salt water to force out any insects in the cauliflower. After soaking, wash it well in fresh water and boil quickly until tender, and serve with white sauce.

CELERY (ITALIAN).

2 heads of celery, ½ pint of milk, 1 oz. of butter, 1 egg, 1 cupful of breadcrumbs, pepper and salt to taste. Cut up the celery into pieces, boil it in water for 10 minutes; drain it and put it into the stewpan with the milk, ½ oz. butter, pepper and salt. Simmer the celery gently until tender, put it aside to cool a little, and add the egg well beaten. Butter a shallow dish, strew it well with some of the breadcrumbs, and pour in the celery, sprinkle the rest of the breadcrumbs over the top, put the butter over it in little bits, and bake the celery until brown.

CELERY (STEAMED) WITH WHITE CHEESE SAUCE.

Prepare the celery as in previous recipe, leaving it in long pieces, and place it in a vegetable steamer, which consists of a large saucepan over which is fitted a perforated top. Add a little pepper and salt, and let the celery steam for 1-1/2 hours. For the sauce you need: 1 pint of milk, 1 oz. of butter, 1 dessertspoonful of Allinson cornflour, 1-1/2 oz. of grated cheese, pepper and salt to taste. Boil the milk with the butter, thicken it with the cornflour smoothed first with a spoonful of water, and last add the grated cheese and seasoning; let the sauce simmer, stirring it until the cheese is dissolved. Have ready some Allinson plain rusks on a flat dish, place the celery on it, pour the sauce over, and serve very hot.

CELERY (STEWED) WITH WHITE SAUCE.

2 or 3 heads of celery (according to quantity required), 2 oz. of butter, 1 dessertspoonful of flour, ½ pint of milk, pepper and salt to taste. Remove the outer hard pieces from the celery, saving them for flavouring soups or sauces; wash well and cut up in pieces about 3 inches long. Set over the fire with ½ pint of water, the butter and seasoning. Let cook gently until the celery is quite tender, which will take about 1 hour; add the thickening and the milk. Let all gently simmer for a few minutes, and serve.

LEEKS.

Remove the coarse part of the green stalks of the leeks. If the leeks are gritty cut them right through and wash them well, and if necessary use a brush to get out the sand. Tie the leeks in bunches and steam them until tender, which will take about 1-1/2 hours. Make a white sauce as for the cauliflower. Put the leeks on pieces of dry toast on a flat dish, pour the sauce over them, and serve.

MUSHROOMS (STEWED).

1 lb. of mushrooms, 1 oz. of butter, ½ pint of water, ½ teaspoonful of herbs, ½ saltspoonful of nutmeg, pepper and salt to taste, juice of ½ a lemon, the yolk of 1 egg, 1 dessertspoonful of Allinson cornflour. Peel and clean the mushrooms, and wash them in water with a dash of vinegar in it. Wipe them dry with a cloth; have the water and butter ready in a saucepan with the herbs, and seasoning. Stew the mushrooms in this for 10 to 15 minutes. Thicken with the cornflour, then stir in the yolk of egg with the lemon juice, and serve.

ONION TORTILLA.

1 lb. of Spanish onions, 1-1/2 oz. of butter or oil, 3 eggs. Melt the butter in a frying-pan, slice the onions, and fry them for 10 or 15

minutes, beat the eggs, add them to the onions, season with pepper and salt, and fry the whole a light brown on both sides.

ONIONS (BRAISED).

2 lbs. of onions, 2 oz. of butter, vege-butter, or oil, pepper and salt to taste. Peel and slice the onions, and fry them a nice brown in the butter. Then add enough water to make gravy, add pepper and salt, and stew the onions for 20 minutes. Eat with wholemeal toast. This is very savoury, and is much liked.

ONIONS (SPANISH) (BAKED).

Peel as many onions as are required, making an incision crossways on the top, and put in a baking-dish with ½ oz. of butter on each large onion, or half that quantity on small ones; dust them over with pepper and salt, and bake them for 3 hours. Keep them covered for 2 hours, and let them brown after that. Baste the onions from time to time with the butter.

SCOTCH OR CURLY KAIL.

Scotch kail is best after there has been frost on it. Wash the kail, and cut away the coarse stalks, boil it for 1-1/2 to 2 hours in a small quantity of water, adding a chopped up onion. Drain it when soft and chop it fine like spinach. Into the saucepan in which the kail was cooked put a piece of butter; melt it, and stir into it 1 tablespoonful of Allinson fine wheatmeal, and brown it very slightly. Then add some of the drained-off kail wafer and stir it smooth with the browned flour. Return the chopped Scotch kail to the saucepan, add pepper and salt to taste; let it cook for a minute, and serve.

SPINACH.

Wash the spinach thoroughly, and set it over the fire in a saucepan without any water, as enough water will boil out of the spinach to cook it. Heat it gently at first, stirring it a few times to prevent it burning, until enough water has boiled out of the spinach to prevent it from catching. Let the spinach cook 20 minutes, then strain it through a colander, pressing the water out with a wooden spoon or plate. Put a piece of butter in the saucepan in which the spinach was cooked; when melted, stir into it a spoonful of Allinson fine wheatmeal, and keep stirring the meal and butter for 1 minute over the fire. Return the spinach to the saucepan, mix it well with the butter and meal, and add as much of the strained-off water as is necessary to moisten it; add pepper and salt to taste, and a little lemon juice. Let the spinach heat well through before serving. Have ready 1 or 2 hard-boiled eggs cut in slices, and decorate the spinach with them. Use 1 oz. of butter, an even tablespoonful of the meal, and the juice of ½ a lemon to 4 lbs. of spinach.

TURNIPS (MASHED).

Peel and wash the turnips, and steam them until tender. Mash them up in a saucepan over the fire, mixing with them 1 oz. of butter. Pile the mashed turnips on a flat dish, and pour a white sauce over them.

EGG COOKERY.

Eggs are a boon to cooks, especially when dishes are wanted quickly. They enter into a great many savoury and sweet dishes, and few cakes are made without them. They can be prepared in a great variety of ways. Eggs are a good food when taken in moderation. As they are a highly nutritious article of food, they should not be indulged in too freely. Eggs contain both muscle and bone-forming material, in fact everything required for building up the organism of the young bird. The chemical composition of hen's and duck's eggs are as follows:—

	Hen's egg.	Duck's egg.
Water	74.22	71.11
Nitrogen	12.55	12.24
Fat	12.11	15.49
Mineral matter	1.12	1.16
	------	------
	100.00	100.00
	======	======

Eggs take a long time to digest if hard boiled. All the fat of the egg is contained in the yolk, but the white of the egg is pure albumen (or nitrogen) and water. Eggs are most easily digested raw or very lightly boiled, and best cooked thus for invalids. The best way of lightly boiling an egg is to put it in boiling water, set the basin or saucepan on the side of the stove, and let it stand just off the boil for five or six minutes. Eggs often crack when they are put into enough boiling water to well cover them, owing to the sudden expansion of the contents. If they are not covered with water there is less danger of them cracking. One can easily tell stale eggs from fresh ones by holding them up to a strong light. A fresh egg looks clear and transparent, whilst stale ones look cloudy and opaque. There are various ways of preserving eggs for the winter; one of the best is by using the Allinson egg preservative. Another very good way is to have stands made with holes which will hold the eggs. Keep these stands in an airy place in a good current of fresh air, and every week turn the eggs, so that one week they stand the pointed end down, next week the rounded end down.

APPLE SOUFFLÉ.

4 eggs, 4 apples, 2 oz. of castor sugar (or more if the apples are very sour), 1 gill of new milk or half milk and half cream, 1 oz. of Allinson cornflour, and the juice of 1 lemon. Pare, cut up, and stew the apples with the sugar and lemon juice until they are reduced to a pulp. Beat them quite smooth, and return them to the stewpan. Smooth the cornflour with the milk, and mix it with the apples, and stir until it boils; then turn the mixture into a basin to cool. Separate the yolks from the whites of the eggs; beat the yolks well, and mix them with the apple mixture. Whisk the whites to a stiff froth, mix them lightly with the rest, and pour the whole into a buttered Soufflé tin. Bake for 20 minutes in a moderately hot oven, and serve at once.

CHEESE SOUFFLÉ.

8 oz. of Parmesan or other good dry, cooking cheese, 4 eggs, 1 oz. of Allinson fine wheatmeal, 1 gill of milk, 1 oz. of butter, mustard, pepper, and salt to taste. Melt the butter in a saucepan, stir in the wheatmeal, season with mustard, pepper, and salt. Pour in the milk, and stir until the mixture is set and comes away from the sides of the saucepan. Turn into a basin, and let the mixture cool. Grate the cheese and stir it in; separate the yolks of the eggs from the whites, and drop the yolks of the eggs, one by one, into the mixture, beating all well. Whip the whites of the eggs to a stiff froth, mix it lightly with the other ingredients; turn the mixture into a buttered Soufflé tin, and bake the Soufflé for 15 minutes.

CHOCOLATE SOUFFLÉ.

5 eggs, 2 oz. of butter, 3 oz. of castor sugar, 2 large bars of chocolate, 6 oz. of the crumb of the bread, and vanilla essence to taste. Cream the butter, and stir into it gradually the yolks

of the eggs, the sugar, and chocolate. Previously soak the bread in milk or water. Squeeze it dry, and add to it the other ingredients. Add vanilla and the whites of the eggs whipped to a stiff froth, and pour the mixture into a buttered pie-dish or cake tin. Bake ¾ of an hour, and serve immediately. If the Soufflé is baked in a cake tin, a serviette should be pinned round it before serving.

CURRIED EGGS.

6 hard-boiled eggs, 1 medium-sized English onion, 1 cooking apple, 1 teaspoonful of curry powder, 1 dessertspoonful of Allinson fine wheatmeal, 1 oz. of butter, and salt to taste. Prepare the onion and apple, chop them very fine, and fry them in the butter in a stewpan until brown. Add ½ pint of water and a little salt. Smooth the curry and wheatmeal with a little cold water, and thicken the sauce with it. Let it simmer for 10 minutes, then rub through a sieve. Return the sauce to the stewpan, shell the eggs, and heat them up in the sauce; serve very hot on a flat dish.

EGG AND CHEESE.

6 eggs, 1 teacupful of milk, thickened with 1 dessertspoonful of Allinson fine wheatmeal, 2 oz. of grated cheese, pepper and salt to taste. Butter a pie-dish, pour into it the thickened milk, break the eggs over it, sprinkle the cheese over them, and season to taste. Bake in a moderate oven until the eggs are just set.

EGG AND CHEESE FONDU.

To each egg ½ its weight in grated cheese and a ½ oz. of butter (if only 1 egg is prepared ½ oz. of butter must be used); mustard, pepper, and salt to taste. Whip up the eggs, add 1 dessertspoonful of water for each egg, as in the previous recipe; mix in the cheese, a little made mustard, and pepper and salt. Heat the butter in a frying-pan or small stewpan. When hot stir in the mixture of egg and cheese. Keep stirring it with a knife, until it becomes a smooth and thickish mass. Put on hot buttered toast, and serve. This is an extremely tasty French dish. The mixture, when cold, is excellent for sandwiches.

EGG AND TOMATO SAUCE.

4 eggs, 1 teacupful of tomato sauce, and ½ oz. of butter. Melt the butter in a flat dish; break the eggs carefully into it without breaking the yolks, and place the dish on the stove until the eggs are set. Heat the tomato sauce, which should be well seasoned, and pour it over the eggs. Serve very hot, with sippets of Allinson wholemeal toast.

EGG AND TOMATO SANDWICHES.

4 eggs, 1 teacupful of tinned tomatoes or ½ lb. fresh ones, pepper and salt, 1 oz. of butter. Melt the butter in a frying-pan, and cook the tomatoes in it until most of the liquid is steamed away; set aside to cool. If fresh tomatoes are used, they should be scalded and skinned before cooking. Beat up the eggs and stir them into the cooled tomatoes, adding seasoning to taste. Stir the eggs and tomatoes with a knife until set, then turn the mixture into a bowl to get cold, and use for sandwiches.

EGG SALAD WITH MAYONNAISE.

1 lb. of cold boiled potatoes, 6 hard-boiled eggs, the juice of ½ a lemon, pepper and salt to taste. Cut the potatoes and eggs into slices, dust them with pepper and salt, add the lemon juice, and mix all well together. Make the mayonnaise as follows; 1-1/2 gills of good salad oil, the yolks of 2 eggs, 1 saltspoonful of

mustard, lemon juice, pepper, and salt to taste. Take a clean cold basin, and place in it the yolks of the eggs beaten up. Drop the oil into them, drop by drop, stirring with a wooden spoon quickly all the time. Great care should be taken, especially in the beginning, as the eggs easily curdle when the oil is stirred in too fast. When the mayonnaise gets very thick add carefully a little lemon juice to thin it down, then add again oil and lemon juice alternately until all the oil is used up. Smooth the mustard with a little lemon juice, and stir it in last of all with sufficient pepper and salt. Taste the mayonnaise, and add lemon juice or seasoning as required. Vinegar may be used instead of lemon juice if the latter is not conveniently had. The mayonnaise should be made in a cold room, as it may curdle if made in a hot room. Should an accident happen, beat up another yolk of egg and start afresh with a little fresh oil, and when going on well stir in, drop by drop, the curdled mayonnaise. Mix part of it with the eggs and potatoes, and pour the rest over the salad; garnish with watercress.

EGG SALMAGUNDI WITH JAM.

4 eggs, 1 oz. of butter, the juice of ½ a lemon, ½ a teacupful of cream or milk, some apricot or other jam. Melt the butter in a frying-pan. Beat the eggs, and mix with them the cream or milk and the lemon juice. Pour the mixture into the butter, and stir it over the fire until it thickens. Stir in some jam, and serve with lady fingers, Allinson rusks, or bread fried in butter.

EGG SAVOURY.

6 hard-boiled eggs, shelled and sliced; in summer use 1 large breakfastcupful of boiled and chopped spinach; in winter Scotch kale prepared the same way; some very thin slices of bread and butter, nutmeg, pepper, and salt to taste, ½ pint of milk, and some butter.

Butter a pie-dish and line it with slices of bread and butter. Spread a layer of spinach and a layer of slices of eggs; dust with nutmeg, pepper, and salt. Repeat the layers, and finish with a layer of bread well buttered. Pour over the whole the milk, and bake the savoury from 20 to 30 minutes, or until brown.

EGGS À LA BONNE FEMME.

4 eggs, 1 Spanish onion, 1 oz. of butter, 1 teaspoonful of vinegar, and 2 tablespoonfuls of breadcrumbs; pepper and salt to taste. Peel and slice the onion, and fry it brown in the butter; add the vinegar and seasoning when done. Spread the onion on a buttered dish, break the eggs over them, dust these with pepper and salt, and sprinkle with breadcrumbs. Place a few bits of butter on the top, and bake until the eggs are set, which will only take a few minutes.

EGGS À LA DUCHESSE.

1 quart of milk, 6 eggs, 1 tablespoonful of Allinson cornflour, sugar to taste, a piece of vanilla 2 inches long. Splice the vanilla and let it boil with the milk and sugar; smooth the cornflour with a spoonful of water, thicken the milk with it, and let it cook gently for 2 or 3 minutes; remove the vanilla. Have ready the whites of eggs whipped to a stiff froth, drop it in spoonfuls in the boiling milk; let it simmer for a few minutes until the egg snow has got set, remove the snowballs with a slice, and place them in a glass dish. Let the milk cool a little; beat up the yolks of the eggs, mix them carefully with the milk, taking care not to curdle them; stir the whole over the fire to let the eggs thicken, but do not allow it to boil. Let the mixture cool, pour the custard into the glass dish, but not pouring it over the snow; serve when quite cold. Half the quantity will make a fair dishful.

EGGS AND CABBAGE.

1 large breakfastcupful of cold boiled cabbage, 3 eggs, 1 teacupful of milk, pepper and salt to taste, ½ oz. of butter. Warm the cabbage with the butter and the milk; meanwhile beat up the eggs. Mix all together and season with pepper and salt. Turn the mixture into a shallow buttered pie-dish, and bake for 20 minutes. Any kind of cold vegetables mashed up can be used up this way, and will make a nice side dish for dinner.

EGGS AU GRATIN.

3 hard-boiled eggs, 1-1/2 oz. of grated cheese, 1 oz. of butter, 2 tablespoonfuls of breadcrumbs, a little nutmeg, and pepper and salt to taste. Slice the eggs, place them on a well-buttered flat baking dish, sprinkle them thickly with the grated cheese, and dust with nutmeg, pepper, and salt. Spread the breadcrumbs over the top, and scatter the butter in bits over the breadcrumbs. Bake until the breadcrumbs begin to brown.

FORCEMEAT EGGS.

6 eggs, 1 small English onion, a few leaves of fresh sage, or ½ teaspoonful of dried powdered sage, a few sprigs of Parsley, pepper and salt to taste, and some paste rolled thin, made of 6 oz. of Allinson fine wheatmeal, 2 oz. of butter or vege-butter, and a little cold water. Boil the eggs for 10 minutes, set them in cold water, and take off the shells. Cut them in half lengthways, remove the yolks, and proceed as follows: Chop up the onion very fine with the sage and parsley, and season with pepper and salt. Pound the yolks very fine, and add the onion and herbs; fill the whites of the eggs with the mixture. Put the halves together, enclose them in paste, brush them over with the white of egg, and bake until the pastry is

done, which will take about 15 minutes. Serve with vegetables and sauce.

FRENCH EGGS.

6 hard-boiled eggs, ½ pint of milk, 1 oz. of butter, 1 dessertspoonful of Allinson fine wheatmeal, 1 dessertspoonful of finely chopped parsley, nutmeg, pepper, and salt to taste. Boil the milk with the butter, thicken it with the flour, smoothed previously with a little cold milk; season to taste. When the milk is thickened shell the eggs, cut them into quarters lengthways, and put them into the sauce. Last of all, put in the parsley, and serve with sippets of toast laid in the bottom of the dish.

MUSHROOM AND EGGS.

4 hard-boiled eggs, ¼ lb. of mushrooms, 1 teaspoonful of parsley chopped very fine, 1 oz. of butter, pepper and salt. Stew the mushrooms in the butter, and season well; chop up the eggs and mix them with the mushrooms, adding the parsley; heat all well through, and serve on sippets of toast.

MUSHROOM SOUFFLÉ.

4 eggs, 1 oz. of Allinson fine wheatmeal, 1 oz. of butter, 6 oz. of mushrooms, pepper and salt to taste. Peel, wash, and cut in small pieces the mushrooms, and stew them in ¾ of a teacupful of water. When the mushrooms have stewed 10 minutes, drain off the liquid, which should be a teacupful. Melt the butter in a little saucepan, stir into it the wheatmeal, and when this is well mixed with the butter, add the mushroom liquor, stirring the mixture well until quite smooth and thick and coming away from the sides of the saucepan. Then stir in the mushrooms, and turn all into a basin and let it cool a little. Separate the yolks from the whites

of the eggs, and stir each yolk separately into the mixture in the basin. Season to taste. Whip up the whites of the eggs to a stiff froth, and mix them lightly with the rest. Turn the mixture into a buttered pie-dish or Soufflé tin, and bake the Soufflé 15 minutes.

POACHED EGGS.

Unless an egg-poacher is used, eggs are best poached in a large frying-pan nearly filled with water. A little vinegar and salt should be added to the water, as the eggs will then set more quickly. Each egg should first be broken into a separate cup, and then slipped into the rapidly boiling water; cover them up and allow them to boil only just long enough to have the whites set, which will take about 2 minutes. Quite newly laid eggs take a little longer. Have ready hot buttered toast, remove the eggs from the water with an egg-slice, and slip them on the toast. Always have plates and dishes very hot for all kinds of egg dishes. Poached eggs are also a very nice accompaniment to vegetables, like spinach, Scotch kale, &c., when they are served laid on the vegetables.

POTATO SOUFFLÉ.

2 oz. of butter, 4 eggs, ¼ lb. of castor sugar, ½ oz. of ground almonds (half bitter and half sweet), 6 oz. of cold boiled and grated potatoes, and 1-1/2 oz. of sifted breadcrumbs. Cream the butter in a basin, which is done by stirring it round the sides of the basin until soft and creamy, when it will make a slight crackling noise. Stir in the yolks of the eggs, the sugar, and almonds; beat for 10 minutes, then stir in the potatoes and breadcrumbs, and last of all the whites of the eggs whipped to a stiff froth. Turn the mixture into a well-buttered dish, and bake in a moderately hot oven from ¾ of an hour to 1 hour.

RATAFIA SOUFFLÉ.

6 eggs, 2 oz. of Allinson fine wheatmeal, 2 oz. of butter, 2 oz. of castor sugar, the grated rind of ½ lemon, ½ pint of milk, 3 oz. of ratafias. Melt the butter in a saucepan, stir in the flour, mix well, and then add the milk, stirring all until the mixture is quite smooth and thick and comes away from the sides of the saucepan. Let it cool a little, then stir in the yolks of the eggs well beaten, the lemon rind, the sugar, and lastly, the whites of the eggs whipped to a stiff froth. Turn the mixture into a buttered pie-dish or cake tin, with alternate layers of ratafias. Bake from ½ an hour to ¾ of an hour in a moderately hot oven, and serve immediately with stewed fruit.

RICE SOUFFLÉ.

6 eggs, 2 oz. of rice, 1 pint of milk, sugar to taste, vanilla essence or the peel of ½ a lemon, and 1 oz. of butter. Stew the rice in the milk with the butter, sugar, and the lemon peel, if the latter is used for flavouring. When the rice is tender remove the peel; or flavour with vanilla essence, and let all cool. Separate the yolks of the eggs from the whites, and beat each separately into the rice for 2 or 3 minutes. Whip the whites of the eggs to a stiff froth, and stir them lightly into the mixture. Have ready a buttered Soufflé tin, pour the mixture into it, and bake the Soufflé for 20 minutes in a hot oven. Sprinkle with castor sugar, and serve at once.

SAVOURY CREAMED EGGS.

To each egg take 2 tablespoonfuls of cream or milk, a little chopped parsley, nutmeg, pepper, and salt to taste, and a slice of hot buttered toast. Butter the cups as in the last recipe, sprinkle well with parsley, beat up the eggs, season with nutmeg, pepper, and salt, and proceed as in "Sweet Creamed Eggs." Serve hot.

SAVOURY SOUFFLÉ.

4 eggs, 1 oz. Allinson fine wheatmeal, 1 gill of milk, 1 tablespoonful of finely chopped parsley, 1 dessertspoonful of finely minced spring onions, 1 oz. of butter, pepper and salt to taste. Proceed as in Cheese Soufflé, adding (instead of cheese) the parsley and onion.

SCALLOPED EGGS.

½ dozen hard-boiled eggs, ½ pint of milk, 1 dessertspoonful of Allinson fine wheatmeal, 1 oz. of cheese, 3 tablespoonfuls of brown breadcrumbs, and 1 oz. of butter. Shell and quarter the eggs; grease a shallow dish with part of the butter, and put the eggs in it. Make a thick sauce of the milk, wheatmeal, and cheese, adding seasoning to taste. Pour it over the eggs, cover with breadcrumbs; cut the rest of the butter in little pieces, and scatter them over the breadcrumbs. Bake till nicely browned.

SCOTCH EGGS.

5 hard-boiled eggs, 1 breakfastcupful of Allinson breadcrumbs, 1 Spanish onion, 1 teaspoonful of powdered sage, 1 dessertspoonful of finely chopped parsley, 1 egg, 1 oz. of butter, pepper and salt to taste, some oil, vege-butter, or butter for frying. Grate the onion, melt the butter, beat up the eggs, and mix them together with the breadcrumbs, herbs, and seasoning. Beat the forcemeat smooth, shell the eggs, cover them completely with a thick layer of forcemeat, and fry them a nice brown. Serve with brown gravy.

SPINACH TORTILLA.

4 eggs, 1 oz. of butter, a teacupful of boiled chopped spinach, lemon juice and pepper and salt to taste. Sprinkle the lemon juice over the spinach, and season well with pepper and salt, and fry it lightly in the butter. Beat the eggs and pour them into the mixture, let the tortilla set, then turn it with a plate, and set the other side. Serve hot.

STIRRED EGGS ON TOAST.

4 eggs, 1 oz. of butter, pepper and salt, 3 slices of hot buttered toast. Whip the eggs up well, add a dessertspoonful of water for each egg, and pepper and salt to taste. Heat the butter in a frying-pan, stir in the eggs over a mild fire. Keep stirring the mixture with a knife, removing the egg which sets round the sides and on the bottom of the frying-pan, and take the mixture from the fire directly it gets uniformly thick. It should not be allowed to cook until hard. Place the stirred eggs on the toast, and serve on a very hot dish. This quantity will suffice for 3 persons.

STUFFED EGGS.

4 hard-boiled eggs, 8 Spanish olives, ½ oz. of butter, pepper and salt to taste. Halve the eggs lengthway, and carefully remove the yolks. Pound these well, and mix them with the olives, which should be previously stoned and minced fine; add the butter and pepper and salt, and mix all well. Fill the whites of the eggs with the mixture. Pour some thick white sauce, flavoured with grated cheese, on a hot dish, and place the eggs on it. Serve hot.

SWEET CREAMED EGGS.

To each egg allow 2 tablespoonfuls of cream, or new milk, 1 teaspoonful of strawberry or raspberry and currant jam, 1 thin slice of buttered toast, sugar and vanilla to taste.

Butter as many cups as eggs, reckoning 1 egg for each person. Place the jam in the centre of the cup; beat up the eggs with the cream or milk, sugar and vanilla, and divide the mixture into the cups. Cover each cup with buttered paper, stand the cups in a stew-pan with boiling water, which should reach only half-way up the cups, and steam the eggs until they are set—time from 8 to 10 minutes. Turn the eggs out on the buttered toast, and serve hot or cold.

SWISS EGGS.

4 eggs, 3 oz. of Gruyère cheese, 1 oz. of butter, 1 teaspoonful of finely chopped parsley, pepper and salt to taste. Spread the butter on a flat baking dish; lay on it some very thin slices of the cheese. On these break the eggs, keeping the yolks whole; grate the rest of the cheese, mix it with the parsley; strew this over the eggs, and bake them in a quick oven for 5 to 7 minutes.

TARRAGON EGGS.

4 hard-boiled eggs, ½ pint white sauce, 1 teaspoonful chopped tarragon, 1 tablespoonful tarragon vinegar, 2 yolks of eggs. Boil the eggs for 7 minutes, and cut them into slices. Lay them in a buttered pie-dish, have ready the sauce hot, and mix it into yolks, tarragon, and tarragon vinegar. Pour over the eggs, and bake for 10 minutes; serve with fried croûtons round.

TOMATO EGGS.

To each egg take 2 tablespoonfuls of tomato juice, which has been strained through a sieve; pepper and salt to taste. Batter a cup for each egg. Beat up the eggs, mix them with the tomato juice, season to taste, and divide into the buttered cups. Cover each cup with buttered paper, place them in a saucepan with boiling water, and steam the eggs for 10 minutes. Serve the eggs on buttered Allinson wholemeal toast.

TOMATO SOUFFLÉ.

4 eggs, 1 oz. of Allinson fine wheatmeal, ¼ lb. of fresh tomatoes or a teacupful of tinned tomato, 1 oz. of butter, 1 clove of garlic or 2 shalots, pepper and salt to taste. Pulp the tomatoes through a sieve. Rub the garlic round a small saucepan, and melt the butter, in it; or chop up very finely the shalots, and mix them with the butter. When the butter is hot, stir in the wheatmeal, then the tomato pulp, and stir until the mixture is thickened and comes away from the sides of the pan, then proceed as before, stirring in one yolk after the other; season with pepper and salt, whip up the whites of the eggs, stir them with the other ingredients, pour into a buttered Soufflé pan, and bake 15 minutes.

WATER EGGS.

4 eggs, 1-1/2 oz. of sugar, the rind and juice of ½ a lemon. Boil the sugar and lemon rind and juice in ½ pint of water for 15 minutes. Beat the eggs well, and add to them the sweetened water. Strain the mixture through a sieve into the dish in which it is to be served, place it in a larger dish with boiling water in a moderately hot oven, and bake until set. Serve hot or cold.

SALADS

These wholesome dishes are not used sufficiently by English people, for very few know the value of them. All may use these foods with benefit, and two dinners each week of them with Allinson wholemeal bread will prevent many a serious illness. They are natural food in a plain state, and supply the system with vegetable salts and acids in the best form. In winter, salads may be made with endive, mustard and cress, watercress, round lettuces, celery, or celery root, or even finely cut raw red or white cabbage; pepper, salt, oil, and vinegar are added as above. As a second course, milk or bread pudding. Salads are invaluable in cases of gout, rheumatism, gallstones, stone in the kidney or bladder, and in a gravelly condition of the water and impure condition of the system.

ARTICHOKE SALAD.

Boil potatoes and artichokes separately, cut into slices; mix, add pepper, salt, oil, and vinegar; eat with Allinson wholemeal bread.

CAULIFLOWER SALAD.

A medium-sized boiled cauliflower, 3 boiled potatoes, juice of ½ a lemon, 2 or 3 tablespoonfuls of oil. Cut up finely the cauliflower and potatoes when cold, mix well with the dressing, and pepper and salt to taste. A little mayonnaise is an improvement, but makes it rich.

CHEESE SALAD.

Put some finely shredded lettuce in a glass dish, and over this put some young sliced onions, some mustard and cress, a layer of sliced tomatoes, and two hard-boiled eggs, also sliced. Add salt and pepper, and then over all put a nice layer of grated cheese. Serve with a dressing composed of equal parts of cream, salad oil, and vinegar, into which had been smoothly mixed a little mustard.

CUCUMBER SALAD.

Peel and slice a cucumber, mix together ½ a teaspoonful of salt, ¼ of a teaspoonful of white pepper, and 2 tablespoonfuls of olive oil, stir it well together, then add very gradually 1 tablespoonful of vinegar, stirring it all the time. Put the sliced cucumber into a salad dish, and garnish it with nasturtium leaves and flowers.

ONION SALAD.

1 large boiled Spanish onion, 3 large boiled potatoes, 1 teaspoonful of parsley, pepper and salt to taste, juice of 1 lemon, 2 or 3 tablespoonfuls of olive oil. Slice the onion and potatoes when quite cold, mix well together with the parsley and pepper and salt; add the lemon juice and oil, and mix well once more.

EGG MAYONNAISE.

4 medium-sized cold boiled potatoes, 6 hard-boiled eggs, 1 bunch of watercress, some mayonnaise. Slice the potatoes, and quarter the eggs. Arrange them in a dish, sprinkling pepper and salt in between; mix pieces of watercress with the eggs and tomatoes, pour over the mayonnaise, and garnish with more watercress.

POTATO SALAD (1).

Boil potatoes that are firm and waxy when cooked, and cut them in slices; let them soak in ½ gill of water, grate a small onion and mix it with these; add pepper, salt, vinegar, and oil to taste. The quantity of oil should be about three times the amount of the vinegar used. Eat with Allinson wholemeal bread.

POTATO SALAD (2).

1 lb. of cold boiled potatoes, 1 small beetroot, some spring onions, olives, 4 tablespoonfuls of vinegar, 2 of salad oil, a little tarragon vinegar,

salt, pepper, minced parsley. Cut the potatoes in small pieces, put these into a salad bowl, cut up the onions and olives, and add them to the potatoes. Mix the vinegar, oil, tarragon vinegar, salt, and pepper well together, pour it into the salad bowl, and stir it well. Garnish with beetroot and parsley.

SPANISH SALAD.

Put into the centre of the bowl some cold dressed French beans or scarlet runners, and before serving pour over some good mayonnaise. Garnish the beans with three tomatoes cut in slices and arranged in a circle one overlapping the other.

SUMMER SALAD.

1 large lettuce, 1 head endive, mustard and cress, watercress, 2 spring onions, 2 tomatoes, two hard-boiled eggs. Shred the lettuce, endive, onions, tomatoes, and cress, place in a salad bowl with mayonnaise dressing, decorate with slices of egg and tomato and tufts of cress.

SUMMER SALADS.

These are made from mixtures of lettuce, spring onions, cucumber, tomatoes, or any other raw or cooked green foods, pepper, salt, oil, and vinegar. Cold green peas, French beans, carrots, turnips, and lettuce make a good cold salad for the summer.

WINTER SALAD.

Cut up 1 lb. of cold boiled potatoes, grate fine 1 onion and mix with these, add watercress, or mustard and cress, and boiled and sliced beetroot; flavour with pepper, salt, oil, and vinegar as above. Hard-boiled eggs may be cut into slices and added, and sliced apples or pieces of orange may be advantageously mixed with the other ingredients.

When oranges are added to a salad the onion must be left out.

POTATO COOKERY

POTATO BIRD'S NEST.

A plateful of mashed potatoes, 2 lbs. of spinach well cooked and chopped, 3 hard-boiled eggs, 1 oz. of butter. Fry the mashed potatoes a nice brown in the butter, then place it on a dish in the shape of a ring. Inside this spread the spinach, and place the eggs, shelled, on the top of this. Serve as hot as possible.

POTATO CAKES

3 fair-sized potatoes, 1 egg, 2 tablespoonfuls of Allinson fine wheatmeal, pepper and salt to taste, and a pinch of nutmeg. Peel, wash, and grate the raw potatoes; beat up the egg and mix it with the potatoes, flour, and seasoning. Beat all well together, and fry the mixture like pancakes in oil or butter.

POTATO CHEESE.

6 oz. of mashed potatoes, 2 lemons, 6 oz. of sugar, 2 oz. of butter. Grate the rind of the lemons and pound it well with the sugar in a mortar, add the potatoes very finely mashed; oil the butter and mix this and the lemon juice with the rest of the ingredients; when all is very thoroughly mixed, fill the mixture in a jar and keep closely covered.

POTATO CHEESECAKES.

1 lb. of mashed potatoes, 4 oz. of grated cheese, 1 oz. of butter, 2 eggs, some bread raspings, 2 tablespoonfuls of Allinson fine wheatmeal, ½ a teaspoonful of mustard, pepper and salt to taste. Melt the butter and mix it with the mashed potatoes, add the cheese, flour, seasoning, mustard, and 1 of the eggs well beaten. Mix all well, and form the mixture into cakes. Beat up the second egg, turn the cakes into the beaten egg and raspings, and fry them in oil or butter until brown. Serve with tomato sauce and green vegetables.

POTATO CROQUETTES.

½ lb. of hot mashed potatoes, the yolks of 2 eggs, ½ a saltspoonful of nutmeg, pepper and salt, 1 whole egg, raspings, some Allinson nut-oil or butter for frying. Beat the potatoes well with the yolks of the eggs and the seasoning; form the mixture into balls; beat the egg well, roll the balls in the egg and breadcrumbs, and fry a nice brown.

POTATO PUDDING.

1 lb. of potatoes well mashed, 1 oz. of butter, 3 eggs, 1-1/2 oz. of sugar, the rind and juice of ½ a lemon, 1 gill of milk. Beat the butter, mix it with the mashed potatoes, add the eggs well beaten, also the other ingredients, turn the mixture into a buttered pie-dish, and bake it ½ hour.

POTATO PUFF.

1 pint of mashed potatoes, 2 oz. of butter, 3 eggs, ½ pint of milk, ½ a saltspoonful of nutmeg, pepper and salt to taste, and a dessertspoonful of finely chopped parsley. Beat the butter with a fork until it creams, mix the potatoes with the butter, whip the yolks of the eggs well with the milk, and stir in the other

ingredients. Add the nutmeg, parsley, and seasoning, and last of all the whites of the eggs, beaten to a stiff froth. The potatoes, butter, eggs, and milk should be well beaten separately before being used, as the success of the dish depends on this. Turn the mixture into a buttered pie-dish, and bake it for 1 hour in a hot oven.

POTATO ROLLS (BAKED).

2 lbs. of cold mashed potatoes, 1 boiled Spanish onion, 1 oz. of butter, the yolk of 1 egg, a little nutmeg, pepper and salt to taste, and a teaspoonful of powdered thyme. Chop up the onion fine, and mix it with the mashed potatoes. Warm the butter until melted, and add this, the yolk of egg, and the thyme. Mix all well, make the mixture into little rolls 3 inches long, brush them over with a pastry brush dipped in Allinson nut-oil or hot butter and bake them on a floured tin until brown, which will take from 10 to 20 minutes. Serve with brown sauce and vegetables.

POTATO ROLLS (Spanish).

3 teacupfuls of mashed potatoes, 3 tablespoonfuls of Allinson fine wheatmeal, 18 olives, 1 egg well beaten; seasoning to taste. Stone the olives and chop them up fine, mix the meal, mashed potato, olive, and egg well together, season with pepper and salt; add a little milk if necessary, make the mixture into rolls, and proceed as in "Potato Rolls."

POTATO SALAD (1).

4 medium-sized cold boiled potatoes, 1 small onion minced very fine, 1 dessertspoonful of finely chopped parsley, oil and lemon juice, pepper and salt to taste. Slice the potatoes, let them soak with 3 tablespoonfuls of water, mix them with the onion and parsley, and dress

like any other salad. Any good salad dressing may be used.

POTATO SALAD (2).

1-1/2 pints of mashed potatoes, 2 hard-boiled eggs, 2 tablespoonfuls of Allinson salad oil, ½ a teacupful of milk, 1 teaspoonful of mustard, pepper, salt, and lemon juice to taste. Make a dressing of the oil, milk, mustard, and seasoning. Mash the yolks of the eggs and mix them with the lemon juice, and add this to the dressing. Chop the whites of the eggs up fine. Mix the mashed potatoes, dressing, and chopped whites of eggs well together. Turn the mixture into a salad bowl or glass dish, and garnish with parsley or watercress and beetroot.

POTATO SALAD (MASHED).

½ pint of mashed potatoes, 2 hard-boiled eggs, 2 tablespoonfuls of Allinson salad oil, 1 dessertspoonful of sugar, 1 teaspoonful of mustard, pepper and salt to taste, 2 tablespoonfuls of lemon juice and seasoning; mash the yolks of the eggs quite fine and mix them smooth with the lemon juice, and add this to the dressing. Chop the whites of the eggs up very fine, mix all together; turn the mixture smoothly into a salad bowl or glass dish, and garnish with watercress and beetroot.

POTATO SAUSAGES.

1 pint of mashed potato, 2 eggs well beaten, 1 breakfastcupful of breadcrumbs, 2 oz. of butter (or Allinson nut-oil), ½ a saltspoonful of nutmeg, pepper and salt. Mash the potatoes well with one of the eggs, add seasoning, form the mixture into sausages, roll them in egg and breadcrumbs, and fry them brown.

POTATO SNOW (a Pretty Dish).

1-1/2 lbs. of potatoes, 3 hard-boiled eggs, 1 small beetroot. Boil the potatoes till tender, pass them through a potato masher into a hot dish, letting the mashed potato fall lightly, and piling it up high. Slice the eggs and beetroot, and arrange alternate slices of egg and beetroot round the base of the potato snow. Brown the top with a salamander, or, if such is not handy, with a coal-shovel made red hot.

POTATO SURPRISE.

1 pint of mashed potatoes, 1 oz. of butter, 4 tomatoes, pepper and salt, 1 tablespoonful of finely chopped parsley. Mix the butter well with the mashed potatoes, season with a little pepper and salt. Butter 8 patty pans and line them with a thick layer of potato; place ½ a tomato in each, with a little of the parsley and a dusting of pepper and salt. Cover with mashed potatoes, and brown the patties in the oven.

POTATO WITH CHEESE.

1 pint of finely mashed potatoes, ½ oz. of butter, 3 oz. of grated cheese, a little nutmeg, pepper and salt to taste. Mix all well with the seasoning, grease some patty pans, fill them with the mixture, and bake them in a moderate oven until golden brown. Serve with vegetables and any savoury sauce.

POTATOES À LA DUCHESSE.

Prepare potatoes as in "Milk Potatoes," leaving out the parsley; beat up, 1 egg with the juice of 1 lemon, let the potatoes go off the boil, add the egg and lemon juice carefully; re-heat the whole again but do not allow it to boil, to avoid the egg curdling.

POTATOES (BROWNED).

1 pint of mashed potato, 1 large English onion, 1 oz. of butter, pepper and salt. Mince the onion very fine and fry it a golden brown in the butter, mix it well with the mashed potato, and add seasoning to taste; form the mixture into cakes, flour them well, place them in a greased baking tin, with little bits of butter on the top of the cakes, and bake them a nice brown.

POTATOES AND CARROTS.

1-1/2 lbs. of boiled potatoes, ¾ lb. of boiled carrots, 2 eggs, 1 oz. of butter pepper and salt to taste, some Parsley. Mash the potatoes and carrots together, beat the eggs well and mix them with the vegetables, add seasoning; butter a mould, fill it with the mixture, spread the butter on the top, bake the whole for ½ hour, turn out, and garnish with parsley.

POTATOES (CURRIED).

6 good-sized potatoes parboiled, 1 oz. of butter, 1 teaspoonful of curry powder, ¾ pint of milk, 1 dessertspoonful of fine wheatmeal, salt and lemon juice to taste. Slice the potatoes into a saucepan and pour the milk over them; smooth the curry powder with a little water, pour this over the potatoes, and add the butter and seasoning. Let the potatoes cook gently until soft; then thicken with the meal, which should be previously smoothed with a little milk or water. Let all simmer for 2 or 3 minutes; add lemon juice, and serve.

POTATOES (MASHED).

To mash potatoes well they should be drained when soft and steamed dry over the fire; then turn them into a basin and pass them through a potato masher back into the saucepan; add a piece of butter the size of a walnut (or more according to quantity of potatoes), and a little hot milk, and mash all well through over the fire with a wooden spoon, adding hot milk as required until it is a thick, creamy mass.

POTATOES (MASHED)(another way).

1 finely chopped English onion to 1 pound of potatoes, piece of butter the size of a walnut, pepper and salt to taste. Fry the onion a nice brown in the butter, taking care not to burn it. When the potatoes have been passed through the masher back into the saucepan, add the fried onion and seasoning and a little hot milk. Mash all well through, and serve very hot.

POTATOES (MILK).

Boil or steam potatoes in their skins; when soft, peel and slice them. Make a sauce of milk, thickened with Allinson fine wheatmeal, and season with pepper and salt. Let the potatoes simmer in the sauce for 10 minutes. Before serving mix into the sauce a spoonful of finely chopped parsley.

POTATOES (MILK) WITH CAPERS.

1 lb. of potatoes, ¾ pint of milk, 1 tablespoonful of finely chopped capers, 1 teaspoonful of vinegar, pepper and salt to taste, 1 tablespoonful of Allinson wholemeal, boil the potatoes till nearly tender; drain them and cut them in slices. Return them to the saucepan, add the milk and seasoning, and when the milk boils add the wheatmeal. Let all simmer until the potatoes are tender, add the capers and vinegar. Then simmer a few minutes with the capers, and serve.

POTATOES (SAVOURY).

1-1/2 lbs. of small boiled potatoes, 1 oz. of butter, 1 dessertspoonful of finely chopped onion, 3 eggs, 1 dessertspoonful of vinegar, pepper and salt to taste, 1 clove of garlic. Slice the potatoes into the saucepan and let them stew gently for 15 minutes with the butter, onion, and seasoning, shaking them occasionally to prevent burning. Rub the inside of a basin with the garlic, break the eggs into it, beat them well with the vinegar, and pour them over the potatoes, shake the whole well over the fire until thoroughly mixed, and serve.

POTATOES (SCALLOPED).

6 medium-sized boiled potatoes, 2 onions chopped fine, and fried brown, 1 breakfastcupful of milk, 1 oz. of butter, pepper and salt, a little Allinson wholemeal. Slice the potatoes; butter a pie-dish, put into it a layer of potatoes, over this sprinkle pepper and salt, some of the onion, part of the butter, and a little meal. Repeat this until the dish is full, pour the milk over the whole, and bake for 1 hour.

POTATOES (STUFFED) (1).

6 large potatoes, 1-1/2 breakfastcupfuls of breadcrumbs, ½ lb. of grated English onions, 1 teaspoonful of powdered sage, 1 ditto of finely chopped parsley, 1 egg well beaten, piece of butter the size of a walnut, pepper and salt to taste. Halve the potatoes, scoop them out, leaving nearly 1 inch of the inside all round. Make a stuffing of the other ingredients, adding a very little milk it the stuffing should be too dry; fill the potatoes with it, tie the halves together, and bake them until done. Serve with brown sauce.

POTATOES (STUFFED)(2).

6 large potatoes, 1 Spanish onion, 1 large apple, 1 oz. of butter, ½ teaspoonful of allspice, 1 dessertspoonful of sugar, pepper and salt to taste, a cupful of breadcrumbs. Chop the onion and apple fine and stew them (without water) with the butter, allspice, sugar, and seasoning. When quite tender sift in enough breadcrumbs to make a fairly stiff paste. Scoop the potatoes out as in previous recipe, fill them with the mixture, tie, bake the potatoes till tender, and serve them with brown sauce and vegetables.

POTATOES (STUFFED) (3).

6 large boiled potatoes, 1-1/2 ozs. of grated Gruyère or Canadian cheese, 1 egg well beaten, pepper and salt to taste, a piece of butter the size of a walnut. Halve the potatoes as before, scoop them out, leaving ½ inch of potato wall all round. Mash the scooped out potato well up with the cheese, add the egg, butter, and seasoning, also a little milk if necessary; fill the potatoes, tie them together, brush over with a little oiled butter, and bake them 10 to 15 minutes. Serve with vegetables and white sauce.

POTATOES (STUFFED) (4).

6 large boiled potatoes, 1 large English onion, ½ oz. of butter, 1 egg well beaten, pepper and salt to taste. Halve the potatoes as before, scoop out most of the soft part and mash it up. Mince the onion very finely and fry it a nice brown with the best part of the butter, mix all up together, adding the egg and seasoning, fill the potato skins, tie the halves together, brush them over with the rest of the butter (oiled), and put them in the oven until well heated through. Serve with vegetables and brown sauce.

POTATOES (TOASTED).

Cut cold boiled potatoes into slices, brush them over with oiled butter, place them on a gridiron (if not handy, in a wire salad basket), and put it over a clear fire. Brown the slices on both sides.

SAUCES

Flesh-eaters have the gravy of meat to eat with their vegetables, and when they give up the use of flesh they are often at a loss for a good substitute. Sauces may be useful in more ways than one. When not too highly spiced or seasoned they help to prevent thirst, as they supply the system with fluid, and when made with the liquor in which vegetables have been boiled they retain many valuable salts which would otherwise have been lost. When foods are eaten in a natural condition no sauces are required, but when food is changed by cooking many persons require it to be made more appetising, as it is called. The use of sauces is thus seen to be an aid to help down plain and wholesome food, and being fluid they cause the food to be more thoroughly broken up and made into a porridgy mass before it is swallowed. From a health point of view artificial sauces are not good, but if made as I direct very little harm will result.

Brown Gravy, Fried Onion Sauce, or Herb Gravy must be used with great caution, or not at all by those who are troubled with heartburn, acidity, biliousness, or skin eruptions of any kind.

The water in which vegetables (except cabbage or potatoes) have been boiled is better for making sauces than ordinary water.

APPLE SAUCE.

1 lb. of apples, 1 gill of water, 1-1/2 oz. of sugar (or more, according to taste), ½ a teaspoonful of mixed spice. Pare and core the apples, cut them up, and cook them with the water until quite mashed up, add sugar and spice. Rub the apples through a sieve, re-heat, and serve. Can also be served cold.

APRICOT SAUCE.

½ lb. of apricot jam, ½ a teaspoonful of Allinson cornflour. Dilute the jam with ½ pint of water, boil it up and pass it through a sieve; boil the sauce up, and thicken it with the cornflour. Serve hot or cold.

BOILED ONION SAUCE.

This is made as "Wheatmeal Sauce," but plenty of boiled and chopped onions are mixed in it. This goes well with any plain vegetables.

BROWN GRAVY.

Put a tablespoonful of butter or olive oil into a frying-pan or saucepan, make it hot, dredge in a tablespoonful of Allinson fine wheatmeal, brown this, then add boiling water, with pepper and salt to taste. A little mushroom or walnut ketchup may be added it desired. Eat with vegetables or savouries.

BROWN SAUCE (1).

1 oz. of Allinson fine wheatmeal, 1 oz. of butter, the juice of ½ a lemon, a blade of mace, pepper and salt to taste. Melt the butter in a frying-pan over the fire, stir into it the meal, and keep on stirring until it is a brown colour. Stir in gradually enough boiling water to make the sauce of the thickness of cream. Add the lemon juice, the mace, and seasoning, and let the sauce simmer for 20 minutes. Remove the mace, and pour the sauce over

the onions. If the sauce should be lumpy, strain it through a gravy-strainer.

BROWN SAUCE (2).

2 tablespoonfuls of Allinson fine wheatmeal, 1 oz. of butter, 6 eschalots chopped fine, 3 bay leaves, ½ a lemon (peeled) cut in slices, pepper and salt to taste. Brown the meal with the butter; add water enough to make the sauce the thickness of cream; add the eschalots, lemon, bay leaves, and seasoning. Let all simmer 15 to 20 minutes; strain, return the sauce to the saucepan, and boil it up before serving.

CAPER SAUCE.

Leave out the onions, otherwise make as "Wheatmeal Sauce." Add capers, and cook 10 minutes after adding them. This goes very well with plain boiled macaroni, or macaroni batter, or macaroni with turnips, &c.

CHOCOLATE SAUCE.

1 bar of Allinson chocolate, ½ pint of milk, ½ teaspoonful of cornflour, ½ teaspoonful of vanilla essence. Melt the chocolate over the fire with 1 tablespoonful of water, add the milk, and stir well; when it boils add the cornflour and vanilla. Boil the sauce up, and serve.

CURRANT SAUCE (RED & WHITE).

½ pint of both white and red currants, 2 ozs. of sugar, 1 gill of water, ½ a teaspoonful of cornflour. Cook the ingredients for 10 minutes, rub the fruit through a sieve, re-heat it, and thicken the sauce with the cornflour. Serve hot or cold.

CURRY SAUCE (1).

3 English onions, 1 carrot, 1 good cooking apple, 1 teaspoonful of curry powder, ½ oz. of butter, 1 dessertspoonful of Allinson fine wheatmeal, salt to taste. Chop up the onions, carrot, and apple, and stew them in ¾ pint of water until quite tender, adding the curry and salt. When quite soft rub the vegetables well through a sieve; brown the meal in the saucepan in the butter, add the sauce to this, and let it simmer for a few minutes; add a little more water if necessary.

CURRY SAUCE (2).

1 onion, 1 even teaspoonful of curry, ½ pint of water, ½ oz. of butter, 1 teaspoonful of Allinson fine wheatmeal, a little burnt sugar. Grate the onion into the water, add curry, butter, and salt, and let these ingredients cook a few minutes. Thicken the sauce with the meal, and colour with burnt sugar.

CURRY SAUCE (BROWN).

2 tablespoonfuls of Allinson fine wheatmeal, 1 oz. of butter (or oil), 1 teaspoonful of curry powder, 1 English onion chopped fine, 1 good tablespoonful of vinegar, a pinch of mint and sage, and salt to taste. Fry the onions in the butter until nearly brown, add the meal, and brown; add as much water as required to make the sauce the consistency of cream; add the curry, vinegar, and seasoning. Let the whole simmer for 5 to 10 minutes, strain the sauce, return to the saucepan, beat it up, and serve.

EGG CAPER SAUCE.

The same as "Egg Sauce," adding 1 tablespoonful of finely chopped capers before the egg is stirred in, and which should simmer a few minutes.

EGG SAUCE.

¾ pint of half milk and water, 1 egg, 1 teaspoonful of Allinson cornflour, juice of ½ lemon, ½ oz. of butter, pepper and salt. Boil the milk and water, add the butter and seasoning. Thicken the sauce with the cornflour; beat the egg up with the lemon juice. Let the sauce go off the boil; add gradually and gently the egg, taking care not to curdle it. Warm up the sauce again, but do not allow it to boil.

EGG SAUCE WITH SAFFRON.

½ pint of milk and water, 1 egg, 1 teaspoonful of cornflour, a pinch of saffron, pepper and salt to taste. Boil the milk and water with the saffron, and see that the latter dissolves thoroughly. Add seasoning, and thicken with the cornflour; beat up the egg, and after having allowed the sauce to cool a little, add it gradually, taking care not to curdle the sauce. Heat it up, but do not let it boil. To easily dissolve the saffron, it should be dried in the oven and then powdered.

FRENCH SAUCE.

1 oz. of butter, 2 oz. each of carrot, turnip, onion, or eschalots, 1 tablespoonful of vinegar, 1 dessertspoonful of Allinson fine wheatmeal, pepper and salt to taste, a little thyme. Chop the vegetables up fine, and fry them in the butter, adding the thyme. When slightly browned add ¾ pint of water, into which the meal has been rubbed smooth. Stir the sauce until it boils, then add the vinegar and seasoning. Let all simmer for ½ an hour, rub the sauce through a sieve, return it to the saucepan, boil up, and serve.

FRIED ONION SAUCE.

Chop fine an onion, fry, add Allinson fine wheatmeal, and make into a sauce like brown gravy.

HERB SAUCE.

Make like "Brown Gravy," and add mixed herbs a little before serving.

HORSERADISH SAUCE.

½ pint of water, 2 tablespoonfuls of grated horseradish, 1 dessertspoonful of Allinson fine wheatmeal, ½ oz. butter, salt to taste. Boil the water, butter, and horseradish for a few minutes, add salt, and thicken the sauce with the meal rubbed smooth in a little cold water; cook for two minutes, and serve.

MAYONNAISE SAUCE.

½ pint of oil, the yolk of 1 egg, the juice of a lemon, ½ teaspoonful each of mustard, pepper, and salt. Place the yolks in a basin, which should be quite cold; work them smooth with a wooden spoon, add the salt, pepper, and mustard, and mix all well. Stir in the oil very gradually, drop by drop; when the sauce begins to thicken stir in a little of the lemon juice, continue with the oil, and so on alternately until the sauce is finished. Be sure to make it in a cool place, also to stir one way only. It you follow directions the sauce may curdle; should this ever happen, do not waste the curdled sauce, but start afresh with a fresh yolk of egg, stirring in a little fresh oil first, and then adding the curdled mixture.

MILK FROTH SAUCE.

½ pint of milk, 2 eggs, sugar to taste, some essence of vanilla or any other flavouring, 1 teaspoonful of Allinson fine wheatmeal. Mix the milk, eggs, flour, and flavouring, and proceed as in "Orange Froth Sauce."

MINT SAUCE.

1 teacupful of vinegar, 1 teacupful of water, 1 tablespoonful of sugar, 1 heaped-up tablespoonful of finely chopped mint. Mix all the ingredients well, and let the sauce soak at least 1 hour before serving.

MUSTARD SAUCE.

1 good teaspoonful of mustard, 1 dessertspoonful of Allinson fine wheatmeal, 1 oz. of butter, vinegar and salt to taste, 1 teaspoonful of sugar, ½ pint of water. Brown the wheatmeal with the butter in the saucepan, add the mustard, vinegar, sugar, and salt, let all simmer for a few minutes, and then serve.

OLIVE SAUCE.

Make a white sauce, stone and chop 8 Spanish olives, add them to the sauce, and let it cook a few minutes before serving.

ONION SAUCE.

1 large Spanish onion, ½ pint of milk, 1 gill of water, 4 oz. of butter, 1 dessertspoonful of Allinson fine wheatmeal, pepper and salt to taste. Chop the onions up fine, and cook them in the water until tender, add the milk, butter and seasoning. Smooth the meal with a little water, thicken the sauce, let it simmer for five minutes, and serve.

ORANGE FLOWER SAUCE

Make a sweet white sauce, and flavour it with 2 tablespoonfuls of orangeflower water.

ORANGE FROTH SAUCE.

The juice of 2 oranges, 2 eggs, sugar to taste, 1 teaspoonful of white flour (not cornflour), add to the orange juice enough water to make ½ pint of liquid; mix this well with the sugar, the eggs previously beaten, and the flour smoothed with a very little water; put the mixture over the fire in an enamelled saucepan, and whisk it well until quite frothy; do not allow the sauce to boil, as it would then be spoiled. Serve immediately.

ORANGE SAUCE

2 oranges, 4 large lumps of sugar, ½ a teaspoonful of cornflour, some water. Rub the sugar on the rind of one of the oranges until all the yellow part is taken off; take the juice of both the oranges and add it to the sugar. Mix smooth the cornflour in 8 tablespoonfuls of water, add this to the juice when hot, and stir the sauce over the fire until thickened; serve at once.

PARSLEY SAUCE.

This is made as "Wheatmeal Sauce," but some finely chopped parsley is added five minutes before serving.

RASPBERRY FROTH SAUCE.

½ pint of raspberries, 1 gill of water, 2 eggs, sugar to taste, 1 teaspoonful of white flour. Boil the raspberries in the water for 10 minutes, then strain through a cloth or fine hair sieve; add a little more water if the juice is not ½ pint; allow it to get cold, then add the eggs, flour, and sugar, and proceed as for "Orange Froth Sauce." This sauce can be made with any kind of fruit juice.

RATAFIA SAUCE.

3 oz. of ratafias, ½ pint of milk; the yolk of 1 egg. Bruise the ratafias and put them in a stewpan with the milk; let it boil, remove from the fire, beat up the yolk of egg, and when the milk has cooled a little stir it in carefully; stir again over the fire until the sauce has thickened a little, but do not let it boil.

ROSE SAUCE.

Make a sweet white sauce, and flavour with 2 tablespoonfuls of rosewater.

SAVOURY SAUCE.

1 onion, 3 carrots, 1 oz. butter, a teaspoonful of Allinson fine wheatmeal, a little nutmeg, pepper and salt to taste. Chop up the onion and fry it a nice brown; cut up the carrots into small dice, cook them gently in 1 pint of water with the onion and seasoning until quite soft; then rub the sauce through a sieve, return it to the saucepan, heat it up and thicken it with the meal, if necessary.

SORREL SAUCE.

Make a white sauce, and add to it a handful of finely chopped sorrel; let it simmer a few minutes, and serve.

SPICE SAUCE.

Make a sweet white sauce, and add ½ teaspoonful of mixed spice before serving.

TARTARE SAUCE.

1 lb. of mushrooms, 1 small onion, ½ oz. of butter, 1 dessertspoonful of Allinson fine wheatmeal, pepper and salt to taste, juice of ½ a lemon. Cook the mushrooms and onion, chopped fine, in ½ pint of water for 15 minutes; adding the butter and seasoning.

Strain the sauce and return it to the saucepan, thicken it with the meal, add the lemon juice, let it simmer 2 or 3 minutes, and serve.

TOMATO SAUCE (1).

½ a canful of tinned tomatoes or 1 lb. of fresh ones, a tablespoonful of Allinson fine wheatmeal, ½ oz. of butter, pepper and salt to taste. If fresh tomatoes are used, slice them and set them to cook with a breakfastcupful of water. For tinned tomatoes a teacupful of water is sufficient. Let the tomatoes cook gently for 10 minutes, then rub them well through a strainer. Return the liquid to the saucepan, add the butter, pepper, and salt, and when it boils thicken the sauce with the meal, which should he smoothed well with a little cold water. Let the sauce simmer for a minute, and pour it into a warm sauce-boat.

TOMATO SAUCE (2).

Cut up fresh or tinned tomatoes, cook with water and finely chopped onions; when done rub through a sieve, boil up again, thicken with Allinson fine wheatmeal made into a paste with water. Add a little butter, pepper, and salt. Eat with vegetables or savoury dishes.

WHEATMEAL SAUCE.

Mix milk and water together in equal proportions, add a grated onion, and boil; rub a little Allinson fine wheatmeal into a paste with cold water. Mix this with the boiling milk and water, and let it thicken; add a little pepper and salt to taste. Eat this with vegetables.

WHITE SAUCE (1).

¾ pint of milk, 1 dessertspoonful of Allinson fine wheatmeal, sugar to taste. Boil ½ pint of the milk with sugar, mix the meal smooth in the rest of the milk, add this to the boiling milk and keep stirring until the sauce has thickened, cook for 3 to 4 minutes, strain it through a gravy strainer, re-heat, and flavour with vanilla or almond essence.

WHITE SAUCE (2).

½ pint of milk, a dessertspoonful of Allinson cornflour or potato flour, a little vanilla essence, 1 teaspoonful of sugar. Boil the milk, thicken it with the cornflour previously smoothed with a little water, add sugar and vanilla, boil up, and serve with the pudding.

WHITE SAUCE (SAVOURY).

¾ pint of milk, 1 good dessertspoonful of Allinson fine wheatmeal, a small piece of butter, size of a nut, pepper and salt to taste. Bring part of the milk to the boil, mix the meal smooth with the rest, add the butter and seasoning, and thicken the sauce. Let it cook gently a few minutes after adding the meal, and serve.

PUDDINGS

ALMOND PUDDING (1).

4 eggs, 3 oz. of castor sugar, 4 oz. of ground sweet almonds, ½ oz. of ground bitter almonds. Whip the whites of the eggs to a stiff froth, mix them lightly with the well-beaten yolks, add the other ingredients gradually. Have ready a well-buttered pie-dish, pour the mixture in (not filling the dish more than three-quarters full), and bake in a moderately hot oven until a knitting needle pushed

through comes out clean. Turn the pudding out and serve cold.

ALMOND PUDDING (2).

½ lb. of almond paste, ¼ lb. of butter, 2 eggs, 2 tablespoonfuls of sifted sugar, cream, and ratafia flavouring. With a spoonful of water make the ground almonds into a paste, warm the butter, mix the almonds with this, and add the sugar and 2 tablespoonfuls of cream or milk, and the eggs well beaten. Mix well, and butter some cups, half fill them, and bake the puddings for about 20 minutes. Turn them out on a dish, and serve with sweet sauce.

ALMOND RICE.

½ lb. of rice, 2-1/2 pints of milk, 1 oz. of butter, 3 oz. of ground sweet almonds and a dozen bitter ground almonds, sugar to taste, 1 teaspoonful of cinnamon, some raspberry jam. Cook the rice, butter, milk, sugar, and almonds until the rice is quite tender, which will take from 40 to 50 minutes; butter a mould, sift the cinnamon over it evenly, pour in the rice, let it get cold, turn out and serve with sauce made of raspberry jam and water. Dip the mould into hot water for ½ a minute, if the rice will not turn out easily.

APPLE CHARLOTTE.

2 lbs. of cooking apples, 1 teacupful of mixed currants and sultanas, 1 heaped up teaspoonful of ground cinnamon, 2 oz. of blanched and chopped almonds, sugar to taste, Allinson wholemeal bread, and butter. Pare, core, and cut up the apples and set them to cook with 1 teacupful of water. Some apples require much more water than others. When they are soft, add the fruit picked and washed, the cinnamon, and the almonds and sugar. Cut very thin slices of bread and butter, line a

buttered pie-dish with them. Place a layer of apples over the buttered bread, and repeat the layers of bread and apples until the dish is full, finishing with a layer of bread and butter. Bake from ¾ hour to 1 hour.

APRICOT PUDDING.

1 tin of apricots, 6 sponge cakes, ½ pint of milk, 2 eggs. Put the apricots into a saucepan, and let them simmer with a little sugar for ½ an hour; take them off the fire and beat them with a fork. Mix with them the sponge cakes crumbled. Beat the eggs up with milk and pour it on the apricots. Pour the mixture into a wetted mould and bake in a hot oven with a cover over the mould for ½ an hour. Turn out; serve either hot or cold.

BAKED CUSTARD PUDDING.

1 pint of milk, 3 eggs, sugar, vanilla flavouring, nutmeg. Warm the milk, beat up the eggs with the sugar, pour the milk over, and flavour. Have a pie-dish lined at the edge with baked paste, strain the custard into the dish, grate a little nutmeg over the top, and bake in a slow oven for ½ an hour. Serve in the pie-dish with stewed rhubarb.

BARLEY (PEARL) AND APPLE PUDDING.

½ lb. of pearl barley, 1 lb. of apples, 2 oz. of sugar, ¼ oz. of butter, the grated rind of a lemon. Soak the barley overnight, and boil it in 3 pints of water for 3 hours. When quite tender, add the sugar, lemon rind, and the apples pared, cored, and chopped fine. Pour the mixture into a buttered dish, put the butter in bits over the top, and bake for 1 hour.

BATTER JAM PUDDING.

1 pint of milk, 3 oz. of cornflour, 3 oz. of Allinson fine wheatmeal, 2 oz. of butter, 3 eggs, some raspberry or apricot jam. Rub the cornflour and meal smooth with a little of the milk; bring the rest to boil with the butter, and stir into it the smooth paste. Stir the mixture over the fire for about 8 minutes, then turn it into a basin to cool. Beat up the yolks of the eggs and add them to the cooked batter; whip the whites of the eggs to a stiff froth and add them to the rest; butter a pie-dish, pour in a layer of the batter, then spread a layer of jam, and so on, until the dish is full, finishing with the batter, and bake the pudding for ½ an hour.

BATTER PUDDING.

½ lb. of Allinson fine wheatmeal, 1 pint of milk, 3 eggs, 1 dessertspoonful of sugar, 1 teaspoonful of ground cinnamon (or any other flavouring preferred). Beat the eggs well, mix all thoroughly, and bake about ¾ hour.

BELGIAN PUDDING.

Soak a 1d. French roll in ½ pint of boiling milk; for 1 hour, then add ¼ lb. of sultanas, ¼ lb. of currants, 3 oz. of sugar, 4 chopped apples, a little chopped peel, the yolks of 3 eggs, a little grated nutmeg and zest of lemon. Mix in lastly the whites of the 3 eggs whisked to a stiff froth, pour into a mould, and boil for 2 hours. Serve with a sweet sauce.

BIRD-NEST PUDDING.

6 medium-sized apples, 5 eggs, 1 quart of milk, sugar, the rind of ½ a lemon and some almond or vanilla essence. Pare and core the apples, and boil them in 1 pint of water, sweetened with 2 oz. of sugar, and the lemon rind added, until they are beginning to get soft. Remove the apples from the saucepan

and place them in a pie-dish without the syrup. Heat the milk and make a custard with the eggs, well beaten, and the hot milk; sweeten and flavour it to taste, pour the custard over the apples, and bake the pudding until the custard is set.

BREAD AND JAM PUDDING.

Fill a greased pudding basin with slices of Allinson bread, each slice spread thickly with raspberry jam; make a custard by dissolving 1 tablespoonful of cornflour in 1 pint of milk well beaten; boil up and pour this over the jam and bread; let it stand 1 hour; then boil for 1 hour covered with a pudding cloth. Serve either hot or cold, turned out of the basin.

BREAD PUDDING (STEAMED).

¾ lb. of breadcrumbs, 1 wineglassful of rosewater, 1 pint of milk, 3 oz. of ground almonds, sugar to taste, 4 eggs well beaten, 1 oz. of butter (oiled). Mix all the ingredients, and let them soak for ½ an hour. Turn into a buttered mould and steam the pudding for 1-1/2 to 2 hours.

BREAD SOUFFLÉ.

5 oz. of Allinson wholemeal bread, 1 pint of milk, 2 tablespoonfuls of orange or rosewater, sugar to taste, 4 eggs. Soak the bread in the milk until perfectly soft; add sugar and the rose or orange water; beat the mixture up with the yolks of the eggs; beat the whites of the eggs to a stiff froth, and mix them lightly with the rest; pour the whole into a well-buttered pie-dish and bake the Soufflé for ½ an hour in a brisk oven; serve immediately.

BUCKINGHAM PUDDING.

¼ lb. of ratafias, 4 or 5 sponge cakes, 3 eggs, ¾ pint of milk, sugar to taste, vanilla flavouring. Butter a mould, press the ratafias all over it, and lay in the sponge cakes cut in slices; then put in more ratafias and sponge cakes until the mould is almost full. Beat the yolks of the eggs well together and the whites of 2 eggs. Boil the milk and pour it on the eggs, let it cool a little, add sugar and flavouring. Pour into the mould. Cover it with buttered paper and steam for about 1 hour. Turn it out carefully, and serve with jam or sauce round it.

BUN PUDDING.

3 stale 1d. buns, 1-1/2 pints milk, 3 eggs, 2 oz. sugar. Cut the buns in thin slices, put them in a dish, beat the eggs well, add to the milk and sugar, and pour over the buns; cover with a plate, then stand for 2 hours; bake for 1 hour in a moderate oven, or steam for 1-1/2 hours, as preferred; serve with lemon sauce.

CABINET PUDDING (1).

½ lb. of Allinson bread cut in thin slices, eggs and milk as in Bun Pudding, 1 breakfastcupful of currants and sultanas mixed, 1 heaped-up teaspoonful of cinnamon, 2 oz. of butter, 2 oz. of chopped almonds, and sugar to taste. Soak the bread as directed in above recipe, add the fruit, which should be previously well washed, picked, and dried, and the cinnamon, almonds, and sugar. Dissolve part of the butter, add it to the rest of the ingredients, and mix them all well together. Butter a pie-dish with the rest of the butter, and bake the pudding in a moderate oven for 1 hour.

CABINET PUDDING (2).

2 oz. dried cherries, 2 oz. citron peel, 2 oz. ratafias, 8 stale sponge cakes, 1 pint of milk, 4

eggs, well beaten, a few drops of almond essence, and some raspberry jam. Butter a mould and decorate it with the cherries and citron cut into fine strips, break up the sponge cakes and fill the mould with layers of sponge cake, ratafias, and jam. When the mould is nearly full, pour over the mixture the custard of milk and eggs with the flavouring added. Steam the pudding for 1 hour, and serve with sauce.

CABINET PUDDING (3).

Butter a pint pudding mould and decorate it with preserved cherries, then fill the basin with layers of sliced sponge cakes and macaroons, scattering a few cherries between the layers. Make a pint of custard with Allinson custard powder, add to it 2 tablespoonfuls of raisin wine and pour over the cakes, &c., steam the pudding carefully for three-quarters of an hour, taking care not to let the water boil into it; serve with wine sauce.

CANADIAN PUDDING.

To use up cold stiff porridge. Mix the porridge with enough hot milk to make it into a fairly thick batter. Beat up 1 or 2 eggs, 1 egg to a breakfastcupful of the batter, add some jam, stirring it well into the batter, bake 1 hour in a buttered pie-dish.

CARROT PUDDING.

3 large carrots, 3 eggs, ½ pint of milk, 4 oz. of Allinson fine wheatmeal, 2 tablespoonfuls of syrup, 1 teaspoonful of cinnamon. Scrape and grate the carrots, make a batter of the other ingredients, add the grated carrots, pour the mixture into a buttered mould, and steam the pudding for 2-1/2 to 3 hours.

CHOCOLATE ALMOND PUDDING.

½ lb. of ground sweet almonds, 7 oz. of castor sugar, 1 oz. of Allinson cocoa, 8 eggs, the whites beaten up stiffly, 1 dessertspoonful of vanilla essence. Place the yolks of the eggs in the pan, whip them well, add the vanilla essence, the sugar, the almond meal, and the cocoa, beating the mixture all the time; add the whites of the eggs last. Pour the mixture into pie-dishes, taking care not to fill them to the top, and bake the puddings the same way as almond puddings.

CHOCOLATE MOULD.

1 quart of milk, 2 oz. of potato flour, 2 oz. of Allinson fine wheatmeal, 1 heaped-up tablespoonful of cocoa, 1 dessertspoonful of vanilla essence, and sugar to taste. Smooth the potato flour, wheatmeal flour, and cocoa with some of the milk. Add sugar to the rest of the milk, boil it up and thicken it with the smoothed ingredients. Let all simmer for 10 minutes, stir frequently, add the vanilla and mix it well through. Pour the mixture into a wetted mould; turn out when cold, and serve plain, or with cold white sauce.

CHOCOLATE PUDDING.

¼ lb. of grated Allinson chocolate, ¼ lb. of flour, ¼ lb. of sugar, ¼ lb. of butter, 1 pint of milk, 3 eggs. Mix the chocolate, flour, sugar, and butter together. Boil up the milk and stir over the fire until it comes clean from the sides of the pan, then take it out and let it cool. Break the eggs, whisk the whites and yolks separately, first add the yolks to the pudding, and when they are well stirred in, mix in the whites. Put into a buttered basin, and steam for 1 hour. Turn out and serve hot.

CHOCOLATE PUDDING (STEAMED).

Three large sticks of chocolate, 1 pint of milk, 3 eggs, 7 oz. of Allinson fine wheatmeal, piece of vanilla 3 inches long Dissolve the chocolate in ¾ of the pint of milk, with the rest of the milk mix the wholemeal smooth, add it to the boiled chocolate, and stir the mixture over the fire until it detaches from the sides of the saucepan; then remove it from the fire and let it cool a little. Beat up the yolks of the eggs and stir those in, whip the whites to a stiff froth and mix these well through, turn the whole into a buttered mould, and steam the pudding 1-1/2 hours. Serve with white sauce poured round.

CHOCOLATE TRIFLE.

8 sponge cakes, 3 large bars of chocolate, ¼ pint of cream, white of 1 egg, 3 inches of stick vanilla, 3 oz. of almonds blanched and chopped, 2 oz. of ratafia, ½ pint of milk. Break the sponge cakes into pieces, boil the milk and pour it over them; mash them well up with a spoon. Dissolve half the chocolate in a saucepan with 2 tablespoonfuls of water, and flavour it with 1 inch of the vanilla, split; when the chocolate is quite dissolved remove the vanilla. Have ready a wetted mould, put into it a layer of sponge cake, next spread some of the dissolved chocolate, sprinkle with almonds and ratafias, repeat until you finish with a layer of sponge cake. Grate the rest of the chocolate, whip the cream with the whites of eggs, vanilla, and 1 teaspoonful of sifted sugar; sift the chocolate into the whipped cream. Turn the sponge cake mould into a glass dish, spread the chocolate cream over it evenly, and decorate it with almonds.

CHRISTMAS PUDDING (1).

1 lb. raisins (stoned), 1 lb. chopped apples, 1 lb. currants, 1 lb. breadcrumbs, ½ lb. mixed peel, chopped fine, 1 lb. shelled and ground

Brazil nuts, ½ lb. chopped sweet almonds, 1 oz. bitter almonds (ground), 1 lb. sugar, ½ lb. butter, ½ oz. mixed spice, 6 eggs. Wash, pick, and dry the fruit, rub the butter into the breadcrumbs, beat up the eggs, and mix all the ingredients together; if the mixture is too dry, add a little milk. Fill some greased basins with the mixture, and boil the puddings from 8 to 12 hours.

CHRISTMAS PUDDING (2).

12 oz. breadcrumbs, ½ lb. currants, ½ lb. raisins, ½ lb. sweet almonds, 1 doz. bitter almonds, ¾ lb. moist sugar, 3 oz. of butter, 2 oz. candied peel, 8 eggs, 1 teaspoonful of spice, and 1 teacupful of apple sauce. Rub the butter into the breadcrumbs, wash, pick, and dry the fruit, stone the raisins, chop or grind the almonds, beat up the eggs, mixing all well together, at the last stir in the apple sauce. Boil the pudding in a buttered mould for 8 hours, and serve with white sauce.

CHRISTMAS PUDDING (3).

1 lb. each of raisins, currants, sultanas, chopped apples, and Brazil nut kernels; ½ lb. each of moist sugar, wholemeal breadcrumbs, Allinson fine wheatmeal, and sweet almonds and butter; ¼ lb. of mixed peel, ½ oz. of mixed spice, 6 eggs, and some milk. Wash and pick the currants and sultanas; wash and stone the raisins; chop fine the nut kernels, blanch and chop fine the almonds, and cut up fine the mixed peel. Rub the butter into the meal and breadcrumbs. First mix all the dry ingredients, then beat well the eggs and add them. Pour as much milk as is necessary to moisten the mixture sufficiently to work it with a wooden spoon. Have ready buttered pudding basins, nearly fill them with the mixture, cover with pieces of buttered paper, tie pudding cloths over the basins, and boil for 12 hours.

CHRISTMAS PUDDING (4).

This is a plainer pudding, which will agree with those who cannot take rich things. ½ lb. each of raisins, sultanas, currants, sugar, butter, and Brazil nuts. 1 lb. each of wholemeal breadcrumbs, Allinson fine wheatmeal, and grated carrots; 4 beaten-up eggs, ½ oz. of spice, and some milk. Wash and pick the currants and sultanas, wash and stone the raisins, and chop fine the Brazil nuts. Rub the butter into the wholemeal flour, mix all the ingredients together, and add as much milk as is required to moisten the mixture. Fill buttered pudding basins with it, cover with buttered paper, and tie over pudding cloths. Boil the puddings for 8 hours.

COCOA PUDDING.

½ lb. of stale Allinson bread, 1 pint of milk, 1 oz. of butter, 3 oz. of sifted sugar, 1 tablespoonful of Allinson cocoa, 3 eggs, vanilla to taste. Boil the bread in the milk until it is quite soft and mashed up; then add the cocoa, smoothed with a little hot water, the sugar, and vanilla. Let the mixture cool a little, add the yolks of the eggs, well beaten, then beat the whites of the eggs to a stiff froth, add these, mixing all well. Bake the pudding in a buttered dish of an hour.

COCOANUT PUDDING (1).

½ lb. of Allinson bread, 3 eggs, 1 pint of milk, 1 grated fresh cocoanut, its milk, and sugar to taste. Soak the bread as for the savouries, add the cocoanut, the milk of it, and sugar, and mix all well. Butter a pie-dish, pour in the mixture, place a few little pieces of butter on the top, and bake as above.

COCOANUT PUDDING (2).

10 oz. of fresh grated cocoanut, 8 oz. of Allinson breadcrumbs, 4 oz. of stoned muscatels, chopped small, 3 oz. of sugar, 3 eggs, 1 pint of milk. Mix the breadcrumbs, cocoanut; muscatels, sugar, and the butter (oiled); add the yolks of the eggs, well beaten, whip the whites of the eggs to a stiff froth, add these to the mixture just before turning the pudding into a buttered pie-dish; bake until golden brown.

COLLEGE PUDDING.

Twelve sponge fingers, 4 oz. of ratafia biscuits, 2 oz. blanched almonds, 2 oz. of candied fruit, and 1 pint of custard made with Allinson custard powder. Butter thickly a pint and a half pudding basin, decorate the bottom with a few slices of the bright coloured fruits, split the sponge fingers and arrange them round the sides of the basin, letting each one overlap the other and cut the tops level with the basin; break up the remainder of the cakes and mix with the chopped almonds, the ratafias crushed, and the remainder of the candied fruits chopped finely; carefully fill the basin with this mixture, not disturbing the fingers round the edge; prepare 1 pint of custard according to recipe on page 75, and while still hot pour into the basin over the cakes, &c., cover with a plate and put a weight on the top, let stand all night in a cold place; turn out on to a glass dish to serve.

CUSTARD PUDDING.

1 quart of milk, 2 oz. of cornflour, 2 oz. of Allinson fine wheatmeal, sugar to taste, and vanilla or other flavouring. Proceed as for a blancmange; when the ingredients are cooked, let them cool a little, beat up the eggs, and mix them well with the rest, and bake all for 20 or 30 minutes in a moderate oven.

CUSTARD PUDDING WITHOUT EGGS.

One dessertspoonful of flour, one packet of Allinson custard powder, 1 oz. of butter, 1 pint of milk, and sugar to taste. Mix the flour and custard powder to a smooth, thin paste, with a few tablespoonfuls of the milk, boil the rest of the milk with the sugar and butter; when quite boiling pour it into the powder, &c., in the basin, stir briskly, then pour into a greased pie-dish and brown slightly in the oven; before serving decorate the top with some apricot or other jam.

EMPRESS PUDDING.

½ lb. of rice, 2-1/2 pints of milk, the rind of ½ a lemon, 3 eggs, some raspberry and currant jam. Gently cook the rice with the lemon peel in the milk, until quite soft; let it cool a little and mix with it the eggs, well beaten. Butter a cake tin, place a layer of rice into it, spread a layer of jam, and repeat until the tin is full, finishing with the rice. Bake the pudding for ¾ of an hour, turn out, and eat with boiled custard, hot or cold.

FEATHER PUDDING.

A teacupful of Allinson fine wheatmeal, a pinch of salt, ½ a teacupful of sifted sugar, and 2 oz. of butter; whisk well together, and add a teacupful of fresh milk, and 2 well-beaten eggs. Beat steadily for 15 minutes; fill a well-greased tin about three-parts full, and bake in a moderate oven for 35 minutes; serve with apricot sauce poured over and around. To make the sauce, take 1 teacupful of apricot jam, add to it 1 gill of water, make very hot, and rub through a heated gravy strainer over and around the pudding; then serve at once.

FRUIT AND CUSTARD PUDDING.

2 cupfuls of stewed and stoned plums (or the same quantity of any other fruit), 1 pint of milk, 3 eggs, 1 large cupful of fine breadcrumbs, sugar to taste, 1 teaspoonful of ground cinnamon, and 1 oz. of butter. Mix the crumbs and fruit in a bowl, oil the butter and mix it with the other ingredients, adding the sugar and cinnamon; beat up the eggs with the milk, and mix it with the rest of the pudding; have ready a greased pie-dish, pour in the mixture, and bake the pudding until nicely brown.

GIANT SAGO PUDDING.

2 oz. of giant sago, 2 oz. of Allinson fine wheatmeal, 2 oz. of currants, 2 oz. of sultanas, 1 tablespoonful of sugar, 1 quart of milk. Soak the sago in cold water, drain, and cook in a double saucepan, if possible, with 1-1/2 pints of the milk for 2 hours; mix the meal smooth with the rest of the milk, add this, the fruit and sugar, and cook it gently for another 15 minutes: then pour the pudding into a pie-dish, and bake it in the oven until set or slightly brown on the top.

GOLDEN SYRUP PUDDING (1).

½ lb. of golden syrup, 1 teacupful of sago, 1 lb. of Allinson fine wheatmeal, ½ pint of milk, 3 eggs, 2 oz. of citron peel. Soak the sago with the boiling milk until quite soft, adding a little water, if necessary; mix it with the meal and golden syrup into a fairly thick batter; beat up the eggs and mix them well with the other ingredients. Butter a mould, cut and arrange the citron in the bottom of it into a star, pour in the batter, tie a cloth over it, and steam the pudding for 3 hours.

GOLDEN SYRUP PUDDING (2.)

This pudding is very much liked and easily made. 10 oz. of Allinson fine wheatmeal, 3 eggs, 1 pint of milk, ½ lb. of golden syrup. Make a batter with the meal, eggs, and milk; grease a pudding basin, pour into it first the golden syrup, then the batter without mixing them; put over the batter a piece of buttered paper, tie up with a cloth, and steam the pudding in boiling water for 2-1/2 hours, taking care that no water boils into it. If liked, the juice of ½ lemon may be added to the syrup and grated rind put in the batter. Before turning the pudding out, dip the pudding basin in cold water for 1 minute.

GOOSEBERRY SOUFFLÉ.

3 pints of gooseberries, castor sugar to taste, ½ pint of milk, 4 eggs. Stew the gooseberries with ½ a teacupful of water until quite soft, adding sugar to taste; rub the fruit through a coarse sieve and place it into a pie-dish; beat the yolks of the eggs well, mix them with the milk previously heated, and pour them over the gooseberries, mixing all well. Bake the mixture in a moderate oven until set; meanwhile beat the whites of the eggs to a stiff froth, adding a little castor sugar, lay this over the Soufflé' a few minutes before it is quite done, let it set in the oven, and serve quickly.

GREENGAGE SOUFFLÉ.

20 greengages, 4 eggs, 3 tablespoonfuls of ground rice, ½ oz. of butter, ½ pint of milk, ½ a teacupful of water, sugar to taste. Skin and stone the fruit; blanch and drop (or grind) the kernels; gently cook the greengages in the water with the kernels and sugar. When the fruit has been reduced to a pulp mix in gradually the ground rice, which should have been smoothed previously with the milk; add the butter and let the whole mixture boil up;

draw the saucepan from the fire and stir in the yolks of the eggs and then the whites beaten to a stiff froth. Pour the mixture into a well-greased dish, and bake the Soufflé' for ½ an hour in a brisk oven. Serve immediately.

GROUND RICE PUDDING.

1 quart of milk, 5 oz. of ground rice, 1 egg, and any kind of jam. Boil the milk, stir it into the ground rice, previously smoothed with some of the cold milk. Let the mixture cook gently for 5 minutes, stir frequently, draw the saucepan to the side, and when it has ceased to boil add the egg well whipped, and mix well. Pour half of the mixture into a pie-dish, spread a layer of jam over it, then pour the rest of the pudding mixture over the jam, and let it brown lightly in the oven.

HASTY MEAL PUDDING (1).

1 pint of milk, 2 oz. of Allinson fine wheatmeal, sugar to taste, a few drops of almond flavouring, 3 eggs, well beaten, some marmalade or other preserve. Boil the milk and meal as for a blancmange, flavour with the sugar and almond essence; let the mixture cool, add the eggs, spread a layer of marmalade or preserve in the bottom of the pie-dish, pour the mixture over, and bake it from 20 to 30 minutes.

HASTY MEAL PUDDING (2).

1-1/2 pints of milk, 4 oz. of Allinson fine wheatmeal, 1 oz. of butter; some jam or golden syrup. Boil the milk and sift the meal in gradually, stirring all the time; let it cook for 5 or 6 minutes, stirring quickly until it is well cooked and a stiff batter; turn it into a dish, add the butter, and eat the pudding with syrup or jam.

LEMON PUDDING.

1 lb. breadcrumbs, 3 eggs, 3 lemons, 2 oz. of sago, 1 pint of milk, 2 oz. of butter, 8 oz. of sugar. Soak the sago well in the milk over the fire, add the butter, letting it dissolve, and mix with it the breadcrumbs, the sugar, the juice of the 3 lemons, and the grated rind of 2. Beat the eggs well, mix all the ingredients thoroughly, and pour the mixture into 2 well-greased pudding basins; steam the puddings 2 hours, and serve them with stewed fruit or white sauce.

LEMON TRIFLE.

Prepare over night 1 pint of custard made by using 1 dessertspoonful of Allinson cornflour and 2 oz. of sugar to 1 pint of milk; let it boil 1 or 2 minutes and put on one side. Next morning add the strained juice of 2 lemons and beat together for 5 minutes; when it is perfectly smooth pour it over slices of Swiss roll which have been laid close together in a glass dish; let the slices be quite covered with the cream. Stand in a cold place for 2 or 3 hours. Garnish with glacé cherries.

LENTIL FLOUR PUDDING.

3 oz. of lentil flour, 1 pint of milk, 3 oz. of sugar, the rind and juice of ½ lemon, 3 eggs, 1 oz. of butter. Boil the milk, smooth the lentil flour with a little water, and pour the boiling milk gradually over it, mixing the lentils well with the milk. Add the butter, sugar, lemon rind, and juice; when the mixture has cooled a little, add the eggs, well beaten; bake the pudding in a well-greased dish in a moderate oven until quite set.

LONDON PUDDING.

2 oz. of Allinson steam cooked oats (to be obtained from any grocer in 2 lb. boxes), 1 large tablespoonful of sugar, ½ pint of milk, 1 oz. of butter and 1 pint of custard made with Allinson custard powder. Boil the milk with the oats, butter, sugar, cook gently for 15 minutes, then pour into a pie-dish and add to the mixture 1 pint of custard made according to recipe given, stir carefully and bake for 1-1/2 or 2 hours; let it cool for a short time before serving.

N.B.—This is a most delicious pudding.

MACARONI PUDDING (1).

4 oz. of macaroni, 2 pints of milk, butter, sugar, 2 eggs. Break the macaroni in small pieces and boil it for 20 minutes. Drain off all the water, pour in the milk, sugar, and a piece of butter. Boil until the macaroni is quite tender. Let it cool, then add the eggs well beaten up, and a little grated nutmeg. Put the pudding into a pie-dish and bake for ½ hour.

MACARONI PUDDING (2).

3 oz. macaroni, which should be boiled in milk until quite tender, place in a buttered pie-dish, and pour over a pint of custard made with Allinson custard powder, bake for ½ hour and serve either hot or cold.

MALVERN PUDDING.

¾ lb. Allinson breadcrumbs, 2 oz. of butter, 1 pint of red currants, 1 pint of raspberries, 6 oz. of sugar, ½ pint of cream. Butter a pie-dish well, spread a layer of breadcrumbs, then a layer of the fruit, washed, picked, and mixed, some sugar and bits of butter; repeat these layers until the dish is full, finishing with breadcrumbs and butter; bake the pudding for

¾ an hour, turn it into a glass dish, whip the cream, spread it over the pudding, and sift sugar over all.

MARLBOROUGH PUDDING.

½ lb. of Allinson fine wheatmeal, 6 oz. of butter, 4 oz. of sugar, ½ lb. of sultanas, 4 oz. of mixed peel, 2 eggs, a little milk. Beat the butter and sugar to a cream, beat in the eggs one by one until well mixed, sift the flour and lightly stir it into the butter, add a little milk if necessary. Then put in the peel cut in very fine strips and the sultanas. Put into a well-buttered mould, which should be only three-parts full, and steam for 2 hours. Turn out and serve with melted butter sauce.

MELON PUDDING.

1 lb. of Allinson breadcrumbs, 3 apples, 1-1/2 lbs. of melon, 12 cloves, ½ pint of milk, 1 oz. of butter, 3 eggs, sugar to taste. Peel and cut up the apples and melon, and stew the fruit 15 minutes, adding sugar and the cloves tied in muslin. Place a layer of breadcrumbs in a buttered dish, remove the cloves from the fruit, place a layer of fruit over the breadcrumbs, and so on until the dish is full, finishing with a layer of breadcrumbs; beat up the eggs, mix them with the milk, and pour the mixture over the pudding; spread the butter in bits over the top, and bake the pudding 1 hour.

MILK PUDDING.

The general rule for milk puddings is to take 4 oz. of farinaceous food of any kind to 1 quart of milk. The best way to prepare most of these puddings is to let the ingredients gently cook on the top of the stove and then to turn them into a pie-dish to finish them in the oven for 4 hour or a little longer, according to the heat of the oven. Should eggs be added, they should be beaten well, then mixed with the pudding before it goes into the oven. Most farinaceous milk puddings are improved by the use of Allinson fine wheatmeal with the other ingredients. For instance, use 2 oz. of giant sago and 2 oz. of wheatmeal to 1 quart of milk; or for semolina pudding, the same quantities of wheatmeal and semolina; and for vermicelli pudding the same, with sugar and flavouring to taste.

MINCEMEAT PANCAKES.

4 oz. of Allinson fine wheatmeal, ½ pint of milk, 3 eggs, some butter, and some mincemeat. Make the batter, fry the pancakes, and place a spoonful of mincemeat on each pancake, fold them up, and serve with sifted sugar.

NEWCASTLE PUDDING.

½ lb. of candied cherries, 3 eggs, Allinson wholemeal bread and butter in thin slices, sugar to taste, 1 pint of milk, a few drops of almond flavouring. Butter a pudding mould and line it with the cherries, fill it with slices of bread and butter; sweeten the milk to taste, and add the flavouring; beat up the eggs, mix them well with the milk, pour the custard over the bread and butter, let it soak for 1 hour; steam the pudding for 1-1/2 hours, turn out, and serve with any kind of sweet sauce.

NURSERY PUDDING.

½ lb. of Allinson fine wheatmeal, a pinch of salt, 4 oz. of vege-butter, and ½ lb. of sultana raisins. Mix all lightly together, then add 4 cupful of golden syrup, the well-beaten yolks of 2 eggs, and teacupful of milk. Mix again, and finally add the whites of 3 eggs whisked to a firm froth; use to fill a fancy mould, and steam for 3 hours; turn out carefully, and serve with sauce.

OATMEAL PANCAKES.

½ lb. of fine oatmeal, 4 eggs, 1 pint of milk. Make a batter of the ingredients, and fry the pancakes in butter, oil, or vege-butter in the usual way. These are very good, and eat very short. Serve with lemon and castor sugar.

OATMEAL PUDDING.

6 oz. of Allinson breakfast oats, 3 eggs, 2 oz. of soaked sago, 1 gill of milk, 2 oz. of sultanas, 2 oz. of currants, 1 even teaspoonful of cinnamon, sugar to taste, 1 oz. of butter. Mix the Allinson breakfast oats with the soaked sago, add the eggs, well beaten, the fruit, sugar, butter, cinnamon, and milk; stir all well, butter a mould, pour the mixture into it, cover with a cloth, and steam the pudding for 3 hours.

OMELET SOUFFLÉ (1).

4 eggs, 6 macaroons, 1 teaspoonful finely minced citron peel, 1 dessertspoonful of cornflour, and sugar to taste. Separate the whites and yolks of the eggs, crush up finely the macaroons and mix well the yolks of the eggs, the macaroons, citron, cornflour, and sugar, adding 1 tablespoonful of water. Whip the whites to a stiff froth, mix this lightly with the rest of the ingredients, butter a mould, large enough to be only half full when the mixture is turned into it, and bake the Soufflé' in a moderate oven until set and lightly browned. Turn out, sift sugar over it, and serve immediately.

OMELET SOUFFLÉ (2).

6 eggs, 1 teacupful of milk, 1 dessertspoonful of Allinson cornflour, 2 oz. of castor sugar, I tablespoonful of orange water. Mix the yolks of the eggs with the orange water, the sugar and the cornflour (previously smoothed with the milk), stirring the whole for 10 minutes; whip up the whites of the eggs to a very stiff froth, and mix this lightly with the other ingredients; have ready a buttered Soufflé dish, pour the mixture into it, and bake the Soufflé about 20 minutes until it is a golden brown and well risen; sift sugar over it and serve immediately.

ORANGE MARMALADE PUDDING.

¾ lb. of Allinson wholemeal bread, some orange marmalade, 1 pint of milk, 3 eggs, some butter. Butter a mould thoroughly, cut the bread into slices and butter them, then arrange the bread and butter in the mould in layers, spreading each layer with marmalade. When the mould is ¾ full, beat up the eggs with the milk and pour it over the layers; let the whole soak for 1 hour; cover the mould tightly, and steam the pudding for 1-1/2 hours. Dip the mould in cold water for 1 minute before turning it out; serve with white sauce.

ORANGE MOULD.

The juice of 7 oranges, and of 1 lemon, 6 oz. of sugar, 4 eggs and 4 oz. of Allinson cornflour. Add enough water to the fruit juices to make 1 quart of liquid; put 1-1/2 pints of this over the fire with the sugar. With the rest smooth the cornflour and mix with it the eggs, well beaten. When the liquid in the saucepan is near the boil, stir into it the mixture of egg and cornflour; keep stirring the mixture over a gentle fire until it has cooked 5 minutes; turn it into a wetted mould and allow to get cold, then turn out and serve.

ORANGE PUDDING.

4 oranges, 1 pint of milk, 3 eggs, 1 tablespoonful of Allinson cornflour, sugar to taste. Peel and slice the oranges and remove the pips, place the fruit in a pie-dish, and sprinkle with sugar; boil the milk, and thicken it with the cornflour; let the milk cool, beat up the eggs, and add them carefully to the thickened milk, taking care not to do so while it is too hot; pour the custard over the fruit, and bake the pudding in a moderate oven until the custard is set. Serve hot or cold.

OXFORD PUDDING.

½ lb. of Patna rice, ¼ lb. of sultanas, 2 apples, pared, cored, and chopped up, 1 teaspoonful of cinnamon, and sugar to taste. Wash the rice, mix it with the other ingredients, and tie all in a cloth, allowing plenty of room for swelling. Let the pudding boil sharply in plenty of boiling water until the rice is soft; time 1-1/2 hours.

PANCAKE PUDDING.

5 or 6 thin cold pancakes, 3 or 3 stale sponge cakes, some jam, 1 pint of milk, 2 eggs, 2 oz. of Allinson fine wheatmeal, vanilla flavouring. Spread the pancakes with jam, roll them up and cut them across into slices. Butter a mould, form a circle of slices round the bottom of the mould against the sides, overlapping each other, and work these circles right up the mould, fill the centre with the sponge cakes broken into pieces. Make a batter of the meal, milk and eggs, adding vanilla to taste; pour this over the rest and steam the pudding for 1-1/2 hours, turn out, and serve.

PANCAKES.

A ¼ lb. each of white flour and fine Allinson wheatmeal, 4 eggs, 1 pint of milk, a pinch of salt, some butter, oil, or vege-butter for frying. Make a batter of the above ingredients. Put a piece of butter the size of a walnut in the frying-pan, and when boiling pour in enough batter to make a thin pancake. Fry a golden brown, turn it over, and when browned on the other side fold the pancake over from each side and slip it upon a hot dish, and keep hot in the oven while the other pancakes are being fried. The above quantity will make 6 or 7 pancakes.

PANCAKES WITH CURRANTS.

4 oz. of Allinson fine wheatmeal, ½ pint of milk, 3 eggs, 2 oz. of currants, sugar and cinnamon to taste, butter for frying. Make the batter the usual way, pick and wash the currants and add them to the batter. Fry into thin pancakes with vege-butter.

PARADISE PUDDING.

1 teacupful of sago, 1 breakfastcupful of Allinson breadcrumbs, 2 tablespoonfuls of sugar, the grated rind and juice of a lemon, 4 oz. of sultanas, 6 apples chopped small, 1 teaspoonful of cinnamon, and 8 well-beaten eggs. Soak the sago over the fire with as much hot water as it will require to soften it, then mix all the ingredients together. Turn the mixture into a well-buttered mould, and steam the pudding for 2 hours. Serve with sauce.

PLUM PUDDING.

This is a plain pudding which can be eaten instead of Christmas pudding by those who are inclined to be dyspeptic ½ lb. of wholemeal breadcrumbs, ½ lb. of Allinson fine wheatmeal, ½ lb. of raisins, 2 oz. of small sago, 2 oz. of butter, 3 oz. of sugar, 2 eggs, 1 teaspoonful of cinnamon, and some milk. Wash and stone the raisins. Rub the butter into the wheatmeal. Mix together the raisins, butter, wheatmeal, cinnamon, sugar, and breadcrumbs. Boil the sago in ½ pint of milk until soft, adding as much water as the sago will absorb. Mix it with the other ingredients, beat up the eggs, add them, and mix all well. If the mixture is too dry add as much milk as is necessary to moisten all well. Fill a buttered pudding basin with the mixture, tie over with a pudding cloth, and steam 3 hours. Eat with a sweet white sauce.

POOR EPICURE'S PUDDING.

1 pint of milk, a stick of cinnamon (4 inches long), 12 blanched and sliced almonds, the thin rind of 1 lemon, sugar to taste, 3 eggs, some Allinson wholemeal bread, and 2 oz. of butter. Boil the milk with the sugar, cinnamon, and almonds; remove the cinnamon, let the milk cool a little, and then add carefully the eggs well beaten. Pour the mixture into a wide, rather shallow pie-dish. Butter slices of bread on both sides, and cover the pie-dish with these; the bread should be free from crust, and entirely cover the milk. Bake in a moderate oven about 45 minutes.

POPPY-SEED PUDDING.

4 oz. of white poppy-seed, 3 eggs, 3 oz. of sugar, 1-1/2 oz. of butter, 6 oz. of Allinson fine wheatmeal, 2 tablespoonfuls of orange-water, and ½ pint of milk. Scald the poppy-seed with boiling water, drain this on and crush the seed in a pestle and mortar, adding a little of the milk. When the poppy-seed has been crushed fairly fine, add the yolks of the eggs, well beaten, the sugar, meal, butter, orange-water, and the rest of the milk; mix all well, beat the whites of the eggs to a stiff froth, add this to the rest of the mixture, turn all into a buttered pie-dish, and bake the pudding 1-1/2 hours.

PRUNE PUDDING.

1 lb. of prunes or French plums, 4 eggs, 1 pint of milk, 1 teaspoonful of Allinson cornflour, sugar and flavouring to taste. Wash the prunes, remove the stones, and soak the prunes in ½ pint of water over night. Stew them very gently in an enamelled saucepan in the water in which they soaked, and add a little more if needed; when the prunes are quite tender, mash them well with a fork or wooden spoon, and let them cool. Beat the whites of the eggs to a stiff froth, and mix this with the mashed prunes when quite cold. Meanwhile make a custard with the milk, cornflour, and the yolks of eggs, adding sugar and a few drops of almond essence; let it cool. Heap the prunes on a glass dish and pour the custard round, and serve.

PRUNE PUDDING

1 lb. of stoned and stewed prunes, ¾ lb. of thin slices of Allinson bread and butter, 3 eggs, 1 pint of milk, sugar to taste. Grease a pie-dish and line it with a layer of bread and butter, then arrange a layer of prunes, and so alternately until the dish is full, finishing with bread and butter; pour a little prune juice over, beat up the egg in the milk, adding a little sugar if liked. Pour the custard over the mixture, let soak 1 hour, and bake 1 hour. The pudding will be much improved if all the liquid is poured off once or twice, and poured over again.

RICE PUDDING (French).

8 oz. of rice, 1 quart of milk, 2 tablespoonfuls of sugar, 4 eggs, 1 teacupful of fine breadcrumbs, the rind of ½ a lemon; boil the rice in the milk with the sugar and lemon rind; let it gently simmer until quite soft, and until all the milk is absorbed; let the rice cool a little, beat up the yolks of the eggs, and mix them with the rice. Thoroughly butter a

pudding mould, and sprinkle it all over with the breadcrumbs. Beat the whites of the eggs to a stiff froth, mix this well with the rice, and turn the whole gently into the mould, taking care not to displace the breadcrumbs; bake the pudding 1 hour in a moderate oven. It should turn out brown and firm, looking like a cake. Serve with fruit sauce or stewed fruit.

ROLLED WHEAT PUDDING.

4 oz. of Allinson rolled wheat, 1 quart of milk, 1 teacupful of currants and sultanas, a very little sugar. Soak the rolled wheat in water for 1 hour. Set the milk over the fire, when boiling add the wheat from which the water has been strained. Let it cook gently for 1 hour, then add the fruit, turn the mixture into a buttered pie-dish, and bake the pudding from ½ to 1 hour in a moderate oven.

RUSK PUDDING.

6 oz. of Allinson rusks, raspberry jam, 1 pint of milk, 4 eggs, a few drops of almond flavouring. Spread a little jam between every two rusks, and press them together. Arrange them neatly in a buttered mould; beat up the eggs, mix them with the milk, which has been flavoured with almond essence, and pour the custard over the rusks; let them soak for 1 hour, then steam the pudding for ½ an hour, turn out, and serve with white sauce.

SEMOLINA BLANCMANGE.

1-1/2 oz. of semolina, 1 pint of milk, 1 oz. of loaf sugar, yolk of 1 egg, a few drops of essence of lemon. Soak semolina in ¼ pint of the milk for 10 minutes, then stir it into the remainder of the milk, which must be boiling; add sugar, and stir over a clear fire for 20 minutes. Take off and mix in quickly the yolk of an egg beaten up with flavouring. Pour into mould previously dipped in water. Serve cold with stewed fruit or custard.

SEMOLINA PUDDING.

4 oz. of semolina, 1 quart of milk, the rind of ¼ a lemon, 1 tablespoonful of sugar, 2 eggs. Mix the semolina smooth with part of the milk; bring the rest of the milk to the boil with the sugar and Lemon rind; add the semolina, let all cook for 10 minutes, then remove the lemon rind, and set the mixture aside to cool; beat up the eggs, mix them with the boiled semolina when it is fairly cool, pour the mixture into a buttered pie-dish, and bake until a golden colour.

SIMPLE PUDDING.

4 oz. of Allinson fine wheatmeal, ½ pint of milk, 4 eggs, 1 even teaspoonful of powdered cinnamon, sugar to taste. Mix the milk and meal perfectly smooth, add the eggs, well beaten, the sugar and cinnamon. Butter some cups, fill them three-parts full, and bake the mixture until done, that is, when a knitting-needle passed through will come out clean. Serve with custard or milk sauce.

SIMPLE FRUIT PUDDING.

Line a plain mould with some slices (about ¼ inch thick) of Allinson wholemeal bread, from which the crust has been removed. Then fill the dish with any kind of hot stewed fruit, and at once cover it with a layer of bread, gently pressed on to the fruit. When cold, turn out, and serve with either custard or white sauce.

SIMPLE SOUFFLÉ.

½ pint of milk, 4 eggs, 1 tablespoonful of Allinson fine wheatmeal, sugar to taste, lemon rind or vanilla, any kind of jam. Smooth the meal in part of the milk, set the rest over the fire with sugar and a piece of lemon rind or 1-1/2 inch of stick vanilla; when boiling, stir the smoothed meal into it, and let it gently cook for 5 to 8 minutes, stirring all the time; remove from the fire to cool; beat up the yolks of the eggs, and mix them well with the mixture (remove the vanilla or lemon rind), beat up to a stiff froth the whites of the eggs, and mix them with the rest. Spread a layer of jam in a pie-dish, turn the mixture over the jam, and bake the Soufflé' until risen and brown. Serve immediately.

SPANISH PUDDING.

8 sponge cakes, 1 pot of apricot jam, 1 pint of milk, 3 eggs, ½ oz. of butter. Slice the sponge cakes lengthways, grease a mould with the butter; line it neatly with some of the slices of the sponge cakes; press them to the mould to keep them in position. Next spread a layer of apricot jam, and fill the mould with alternate layers of sponge cake and jam. Beat up the yolks of the eggs and mix them with the milk; pour the mixture over the pudding, and bake it in a slow oven until set. Let the pudding get cold, and turn it out carefully. Have ready the whites of the eggs beaten to a stiff froth, with a little sugar; pile the froth over the pudding, and serve with custard.

SPONGE DUMPLINGS.

2 eggs, 1-1/2 gills of milk, 2 oz. of Allinson fine wheatmeal, ½ oz. of butter, mace, pepper, and salt to taste. Separate the yolks from the whites of the eggs; mix the wheatmeal with the milk, adding the whites of the eggs, a little mace, pepper and salt. Stir the mixture over the fire with the butter until it is quite thick and comes away from the saucepan; take the mixture from the fire, and when a little cooled

add the yolks. Cut off lumps with a spoon and drop them into the boiling soup.

STUFFED SWEET ROLLS.

4 Allinson wholemeal rolls, 3 cooking apples, 2 oz. of ground sweet almonds, 4 oz. of macaroons crushed, 2 oz. of currants, picked and washed, 2 eggs, a little milk, cinnamon, 1 oz. of butter, sugar to taste. Halve the rolls lengthways and remove the crumb; soak the crusts for a few minutes in a little cold milk when the stuffing is ready. Pare and core the apples, cook them with 1/3 teacupful of water, ½ oz. of the butter, and 1 tablespoonful of sugar, and mash them up to a pulp with a wooden spoon; then add the currants, almonds, macaroons, 1 egg well beaten, and the yolk of the other. Mix all well, and add some of the breadcrumbs to make the whole into a fairly firm mass. Fill the crusts of the rolls with the mixture, press the two halves of each roll together, place the rolls into a baking tin, sprinkle them with sugar and powdered cinnamon, scatter bits of butter over the crusts, and bake the rolls for ½ hour. Serve with white sauce.

TAPIOCA PUDDING.

1 oz. of tapioca, 1 egg, ½ pint of cold milk, 1 gill of cold water, ¼ oz. of butter, ½ oz. of moist sugar, cinnamon to taste. Put the tapioca into a basin, and cover it with water. Let it soak for 1 hour, until it has absorbed all the water. Add the milk and sugar. Bring to a boil, and simmer till quite soft and clear. Draw to the side of the fire, to cool it a little. Break the egg and beat it slightly; mix well with the tapioca; pour into a greased dish, and bake in a moderate oven until it is a golden colour. Serve either hot or cold.

VANILLA CHESTNUTS (for Dessert).

1 lb. of chestnuts, ½ lb. of sugar, 1 teacupful of water, vanilla to taste. Boil the chestnuts in plenty of water until tender, but not too soft, that they may not break in peeling. Peel them; simmer the sugar and the teacupful of water for 10 minutes, then add the chestnuts. Allow all to cook gently until the syrup browns, add vanilla and remove the chestnuts from the fire; when sufficiently cool, turn the whole into a glass dish.

WHOLEMEAL BANANA PUDDING.

2 teacupfuls of Allinson fine wheatmeal, 3 oz. of sago, 6 bananas, 1 tablespoonful of sugar, 3 eggs, ½ pint of milk. Peel the bananas and mash them with a fork. Soak the sago with ½ pint of water, either in the oven or in a saucepan. Make a batter with the eggs, meal, and milk; add the bananas, sugar, and sago, and mix all smoothly. Turn the mixture into a greased mould and steam the pudding for 2 hours.

WINIFRED PUDDING.

3 oz. of butter, 3 oz. of sugar, 2 eggs, 1 oz. of Allinson breadcrumbs, the juice of 1 lemon, flavouring, puff paste. Beat the butter and sugar to a cream, beat in the eggs one at a time. Pour sufficient boiling milk over the breadcrumbs to soak, and add them to the mixture, add the strained lemon juice and flavouring, and mix well together. Border a pie-dish and line with paste; put in the mixture, and bake for about 30 minutes in a moderate oven. Sift a little white sugar over, and serve hot or cold.

YORKSHIRE PUDDING.

The old-fashioned way of making it is with white flour. Try this way. 4 oz. each of Allinson breakfast oats and Allinson fine wheatmeal, 4 eggs, 1 pint of milk, pepper and salt to taste. Whip the eggs well, and make a batter of the eggs, milk, meal and oats, adding pepper and salt. Pour the mixture into a shallow Yorkshire pudding tin, which has been previously well buttered. Scatter a few bits of butter on the top, and bake the pudding for 1 hour. Serve with baked potatoes, green vegetables, and sauce.

PIES

PIE-CRUSTS.

(1) 1 lb. of Allinson fine wheatmeal, 6 oz. of butter, a little cold water. Rub the butter into the meal, add enough water to the paste to keep it together, mixing it with a knife, roll out and use.

(2) ½ lb. of Allinson fine wheatmeal, ½ lb. of mashed potatoes, 3 oz. of butter, 1 tablespoonful of oil, a little cold milk (about 1 cupful). Mix the meal and mashed potatoes, rub in the butter and the oil, add enough milk to moisten the paste, mixing with a knife only, and roll out as required.

(3) ½ lb. of Allinson fine wheatmeal, 4 eggs, 2 oz. of butter, some milk. Rub the butter into the meal, beat the eggs well, mix them with the meal, adding enough cold milk to make a firm paste, roll out and use.

(4) ½ lb. of Allinson fine wheatmeal, ½ lb. of fine breadcrumbs, 2 eggs, 2 oz. of butter, and a little cold milk. Mix the ingredients as in (3), moisten the paste with milk, and roll it out.

(5) (Puff crust). 1 lb. of Allinson fine wheatmeal, 1 lb. of butter, a little cold water. Rub ½ lb. of butter into the meal, add enough cold water to make a stiff paste, roll it out, spread the paste with some of the other butter, and roll the paste up; roll it out again, spread with more butter, roll up again and repeat about 3 times, until all the butter is used up. Use for pie-crust, &c., and bake in a quick oven.

(6) ½ lb. of Allinson fine wheatmeal, 3 oz. of sago, 1 oz. of butter. Let the sago swell out over the fire with milk and water, mix it with the meal and butter, and roll the paste out and use.

(7) 1 lb. of Allinson fine wheatmeal, 1 gill of cold milk, 5 oz. vege-butter. Rub the butter well into the meal, moisten with the milk (taking a little more than 1 gill if necessary), in the usual way. Roll out and use according to requirements.

TARTS

Special recipes for every kind of fruit tart are not given, as the same rules apply to all. For the crust either of the recipes given for pie-crusts may be used, and the fruit tarts can be made either open, with a bottom crust only, with top and bottom crust, or with a top crust only. When any dried fruit is used, like prunes, dried apricots, apple-rings, &c., these should first be stewed till tender, and sweetened if necessary, and allowed to cool; then place as much of the fruit as is required into your tart, cover it with a crust, and bake until the crust is done. If an open tart is made, only very little juice should be used, as it would make the crust heavy.

Summer fruit, like strawberries, raspberries, currants, cherries, and gooseberries need not be previously cooked. Mix the fruit with the necessary sugar, and it the tart is made with a top crust only, a little water can be added and an egg-cup or a little tea-cup should be placed in the pie-dish upside down to keep up the crust.

BLANCMANGE TARTLETS.

1 pint of milk, 3 oz. of ground rice, 1 teaspoonful of sugar, a few drops of almond essence, any kind of jam preferred. Make a blancmange, of the milk, ground rice, and flavouring; grease some patty pans, fill them with the blancmange mixture, place a spoonful of jam on every tartlet, and bake them 10 minutes.

CHEESECAKES (ALMOND).

3 oz. of sweet ground almonds, ½ oz. bitter ground almonds, 3 oz. castor sugar, 1 egg, 1 dessertspoonful of orange-water. Pound the almonds well together with the orange-water, and the sugar, beat the egg and mix it well with the almonds. Line 8 or 10 little cheesecake tins with a short crust, bake them, fill with the almond mixture, and serve cold.

CHOCOLATE TARTS.

6 oz. of Allinson fine wheatmeal, 2 oz. of butter, 2 oz. of Allinson chocolate (grated), 1 dessertspoonful of sugar, ½ oz. of ground rice, 4 eggs, well beaten, and 1 pint of milk. Mix the milk with the ground rice, add to it the chocolate smoothly and gradually; stir the mixture over the fire until it thickens, let cool a little and stir in the eggs; make the meal and butter into a paste with a little cold water; line a greased plate with it, and pour the cooled

custard into it; bake the tart ½ hour in a moderate oven.

MARLBOROUGH PIE.

6 good-sized apples, 1 oz. of butter, 3 eggs, the juice and rind of 1 lemon, 1 teacupful of milk, sugar to taste, and some paste for crust. Steam or bake the apples till tender and press them through a sieve while hot, add the butter, and let the mixture cool; beat the yolks of the eggs, add to them the milk, sugar, lemon juice and rind, and add all these to the apples and butter; line a dish with paste, fill it with the above mixture, and bake the pie for ½ hour in a quick oven; whip the whites of the eggs stiff, adding a little castor sugar, heap the froth over the pie, and let it set in the oven.

LEMON CREAM (for Cheesecakes).

1 lb. powdered sugar, 6 yolks of eggs, 4 whites of eggs, juice of 8 lemons, grated rind of 2 lemons, ¼ lb. fresh butter. Put the ingredients into a double boiler and stir over a slow fire until the cream is the consistency of honey.

LEMON TART.

1 lemon, 1 breakfastcupful of water, 1 dessertspoonful of cornflour, 2 eggs, 1 oz. of butter, sugar to taste, some short crust made of 4 oz. of Allinson's fine wheatmeal and 1-1/2 oz. of butter. Moisten the cornflour with a little of the water; bring the rest of the water to the boil with the juice and the grated rind of the lemon and sugar. Thicken the mixture with the cornflour; let it simmer for a few minutes, then set aside to cool; beat up the eggs, mix them well through with the rest of the ingredients, line a flat dish or soup-plate with pastry; pour the mixture into this, cover the tart with thin

strips of pastry in diamond shape, and bake the tart ¾ of an hour.

TREACLE TART.

To 1 lb. of golden syrup add 1 breakfastcupful of Allinson breadcrumbs, the grated rind and juice of 1 lemon. Mix well together. Line the tins with short paste. Put about 1 tablespoonful of the mixture in each tin; bake in a quick oven.

BLANCMANGES

BLANCMANGE.

1 quart of milk, 2 oz. of Allinson fine wheatmeal, 2 oz. of Allinson cornflour, 1 oz. of sugar, piece of vanilla 3 inches long, or some vanilla essence. Bring 1-1/2 pints of milk to the boil, adding the vanilla spliced and the sugar; mix the wheatmeal and cornflour smooth with the rest of the milk, add the mixture to the boiling milk, stir all well for 8 to 10 minutes, and then pour it into one or two wetted moulds; when cold, turn out and serve with stewed fruit or jam.

BLANCMANGE (CHOCOLATE).

1 quart of milk, 1 oz. of N.F. cocoa, 2 oz. of Allinson cornflour, 2 oz. of sifted Allinson fine wheatmeal, sugar to taste, 1 good dessertspoonful of vanilla essence. Set the greatest part of the milk over the fire, leaving enough to smooth the cornflour, flour, and cocoa. Mix the cornflour, wheatmeal flour, and cocoa, and smooth it with the cold milk. Stir the mixture into the boiling milk, and let it all simmer for 8 to 10 minutes, stirring very frequently. Add the vanilla essence, stir it well

through, pour the mixture into a wetted mould, and let it get cold. Turn it out, and serve.

BLANCMANGE (LEMON) (a very good Summer Pudding).

1 pint of water, 2 tablespoonfuls of Allinson cornflour, 1 lemon, 2 eggs, sugar to taste. Put the water in an enamel saucepan, and let it boil with the rind of the lemon in it. When boiling, add the cornflour mixed with a little cold water. Allow it all to boil for a few minutes; then add sugar and the juice of a lemon. Have the whites of the eggs beaten to a stiff froth, and beat up well with the mixture; then pour into a mould. Make a little custard to pour over the blancmange—1/2 pint of milk, a little sugar, and essence of lemon; whisk in the yolks of the eggs. This makes an excellent custard.

BLANCMANGE EGGS.

Make a blancmange with 1 pint of milk, 1 oz. of Allinson cornflour, and 1 oz. of Allinson fine wheatmeal. Pierce the ends of 4 or 6 eggs, and let the contents drain away. Rinse the shells with cold water, then fill them with the hot blancmange mixture. When cold gently peel off the shells. Serve on a glass dish nicely arranged with stewed fruit or jam.

ORANGE MOULD (1).

7 oranges, 1 lemon, 4 oz. of cornflour, 4 oz. of sugar, 4 eggs, some water. Take the juice of the oranges and lemon and the grated rind of the latter. Add enough water to the juice to make 1 quart of liquid. Set that over the fire to boil (keeping back a ¼ of a pint for mixing the cornflour smooth), and add the sugar. Separate the yolks of the eggs from the white; beat up the yolks and add them to the cornflour and juice when those are smooth.

When the liquid over the fire boils, stir in the mixture of eggs, cornflour, and juice, and keep all stirring over the fire for 2 minutes. Have ready the whites of the eggs beaten to a stiff froth, mix it lightly with the rest, and pour the mixture into wetted moulds. Turn out when cold and serve when required.

ORANGE MOULD (2).

The juice of 7 oranges and 1 lemon, 6 oz. of sugar, 4 oz. of Allinson cornflour, and 4 eggs. Add enough water to the fruit juice to make 1 quart of liquid. Put 1-1/2 pints of this over the fire with the sugar. When boiling thicken it with the cornflour, which should be smoothed with the rest of the liquid. Stir well over the fire for 5 to 8 minutes; whip up the eggs and stir them carefully into the mixture so as not to curdle them. Pour all into a wetted mould, let it get cold, turn it out, and serve.

CREAMS

APRICOT CREAMS.

1 pint of cream, the whites of 4 eggs, some apricot jam, 2 inches of vanilla pod, 1 dessertspoonful of castor sugar. Split the vanilla, put this and the sugar into the cream; whip this with the whites of eggs until stiff, then remove the vanilla. Place a good teaspoonful of apricot jam in each custard glass, and fill up with whipped cream.

BLACKBERRY CREAM.

1 quart of blackberries, sugar to taste, ½ pint of cream, white of 2 eggs. Mash the fruit gently, put it into a hair-sieve and allow it to drain. Sprinkle the fruit with sugar to make the

juice drain more freely; whip the cream and mix with the juice.

CHOCOLATE CREAM.

1 quart of milk, 6 oz. of Allinson chocolate, 4 eggs, 1 tablespoonful of Allinson corn flour, essence of vanilla, sugar to taste. Dissolve the chocolate in a few tablespoonfuls of water, stirring it over the fire until a thick, smooth paste; add the milk, vanilla, and sugar. When boiling thicken the milk with the cornflour; remove the mixture from the fire to cool slightly, beat the eggs well, stir them into the thickened chocolate very gradually, and stir the whole over the fire, taking care not to allow it to boil When well thickened let the cream cool; serve in custard glasses or poured over sponge cakes or macaroons.

CHOCOLATE CREAM (French) (1).

Use the whites of 3 eggs to 2 large bars of chocolate; vanilla to taste. Break the chocolate in pieces, and melt it in a little enamelled saucepan with very little water; stir it quite smooth, and flavour with Allinson vanilla essence. Set the chocolate aside until quite cold, when it should be a smooth paste, and not too firm. Beat the whites of the eggs to a very stiff froth, and mix the chocolate with it, stirring both well together until the chocolate is well mixed with the froth. It the cream is not found sweet enough, add a little castor sugar. Serve in a glass dish. This is easily made, and very dainty.

CHOCOLATE CREAM (WHIPPED).

2 oz. of Allinson chocolate to ¼ pint of cream, white of 1 egg. Dissolve the chocolate over the fire with 2 tablespoonfuls of water; let it get quite cold, and then mix it with the cream

previously whipped stiff; this will not require any additional sugar.

EGG CREAM.

The yolks of 6 eggs, ½ pint of water, juice of 1 lemon, 2 oz. of sifted sugar, a little cinnamon. Beat up all the ingredients, put the mixture into a saucepan over a sharp fire, and whisk it till quite frothy, taking care not to let it boil; fill into glasses and serve at once.

LEMON CREAM.

The juice of 3 lemons and the rind of 1, 7 eggs, 6 oz. of sugar, 1 dessertspoonful of cornflour. Proceed exactly as in "Orange Cream."

MACAROON CREAM.

Pound 1-1/2 doz. macaroons, place in a bowl, add 1 or 2 spoonfuls of milk, and mix all to a smooth paste. Take a 6d. jar of cream, whip to a stiff froth. Lay a little of the macaroon paste roughly in the bottom of a glass dish, then 1 or 2 spoonfuls of the cream, more paste and cream, then cover with 1 spoonful of cream put on roughly.

ORANGE CREAM.

6 oranges, 1 lemon, 7 eggs, 4 to 6 oz. of sugar (according to taste), 1 dessertspoonful of cornflour, some water. Take the juice of the oranges and the juice and grated rind of the lemon. Add enough water to the fruit juice to make 1-1/2 pints of liquid; let this get hot, adding the sugar to it; mix the cornflour smooth with a spoonful of cold water, and thicken the fruit juice with it, letting it boil up for a minute, set aside and let it cool a little; beat the eggs well, and when the liquid has cooled mix them carefully in with it; return the

whole over a gentle fire, keep stirring continually until the cream thickens, but take care not to let it boil, as this would curdle it. When cold, serve in custard glasses, or in a glass dish poured over macaroons.

RASPBERRY CREAM.

1 quart of raspberries, sugar to taste, ½ pint of cream. Proceed as in "Blackberry Cream."

RUSSIAN CREAM.

Lay 6 sponge cakes on a glass dish, and soak them with any fruit syrup; then add 1 pint of blancmange. When nearly cold cover the top with ratafia biscuits and decorate with angelica and cherries.

STRAWBERRY CREAM.

1 quart of strawberries, sugar to taste, ½ pint of cream. Proceed as in "Blackberry Cream."

SWISS CREAM.

½ pint of cream, ½ pint of milk, 1 tablespoonful of Allinson cornflour, ¼ lb. of macaroons, 2 oz. of ratafias, vanilla, and sugar to taste. Put the cream and milk over the fire, adding a piece of vanilla 2 inches long, and sugar to taste; smooth the cornflour with a tablespoonful of cold milk, mix it with the milk and cream when nearly boiling, stir the mixture over the fire until it has thickened and let it simmer 2 minutes longer, always stirring; remove the vanilla, arrange the macaroons and ratafias on a shallow glass dish, let the cream cool a little, then pour it over the biscuits and serve cold. This makes a delicious dish.

WHIPPED CREAMS.

Quantity of good thick cream according to requirement. The white of 1 egg to ¼ pint. Whip it well with a whisk or fork until it gets quite thick; in hot weather it should be kept on ice or standing in another basin with cold water, as the cream might curdle. Add sugar to taste and whatever flavouring might be desired, this latter giving the cream its name. When whipped cream is used to pour over sweets, &c., flavour it with stick vanilla; a piece 1 inch long is sufficient for ½ pint of cream; it must be split and as much as possible of the little grains in it rubbed into the cream.

CUSTARDS

ALMOND CUSTARD.

1 quart of milk, 6 eggs, 1 dessertspoonful of Allinson cornflour, 1 wineglassful of rosewater, sugar to taste, ½ lb. ground almonds. Boil the milk with the sugar and almonds; smooth the cornflour with the rosewater and stir it into the boiling milk, let it boil up for a minute. Beat up the eggs, leaving out 3 of the whites of the eggs, which are to be beaten to a stiff froth. Let the milk cool a little, then stir in the eggs very gradually, taking care not to curdle them; stir over the fire until the custard is nearly boiling, then let it cool, stirring occasionally; pour it into a glass dish, and pile the whipped whites of the eggs on the top of the custard just before serving.

BAKED APPLE CUSTARD.

8 large apples, moist sugar to taste, half a teacupful of water and the juice of half a lemon, 1 pint of custard made with Allinson custard powder. Peel, cut and core the apples and put into a lined saucepan with the water,

sugar, and lemon juice, stew till tender and rub through a sieve; when cold put the fruit at the bottom of a pie-dish and pour the custard over, grate a little nutmeg over the top, bake lightly, and serve cold.

BAKED CUSTARD.

1 quart of milk, 6 eggs, sugar, and flavouring to taste. Heat the milk until nearly boiling, sweeten it with sugar, and add any kind of flavouring. Whip up the eggs, and mix them carefully with the hot milk. Pour the custard into a buttered pie-dish, and bake it in a moderately hot oven until set. If the milk and eggs are mixed cold and then baked the custard goes watery; it is therefore important to bear in mind that the milk should first be heated. Serve with stewed fruit.

CARAMEL CUSTARD.

1-1/2 pints of milk, 4 eggs, 1 dessertspoonful of sugar, ½ lemon and 4 oz. of castor sugar for caramel. Put the dry castor sugar into an enamelled saucepan and let it melt and turn a rich brown over the fire, stirring all the time. When the sugar is melted and browned stir into it about 2 tablespoonfuls of hot water, and the juice of ½ lemon. Then pour the caramel into a mould or cake-tin, and let it run all round the sides of the tin. Meanwhile heat the milk near boiling-point, and add the vanilla and sugar. Whip up the eggs, stir carefully into them the hot milk, so as not to curdle the eggs. Then pour the custard into the tin on the caramel and stand the tin in a larger tin with hot water, place it in the oven, and bake in a moderately hot oven for about 20 minutes or until the custard is set. Allow it to get cold, turn out, and serve.

CARAMEL CUP CUSTARD (French).

Make the custard as in the recipe for "Cup Custard." Take 4 oz. of castor sugar; put it over a brisk fire in a small enamelled saucepan, keep stirring it until quite melted and a rich brown. Then cautiously add 2 tablespoonfuls of boiling water, taking care not to be scalded by the spluttering sugar. Gradually stir the caramel into the hot custard. Let it cool, and serve in custard glasses.

CUP CUSTARD.

6 whole eggs or 10 yolks of eggs, 1 quart of milk, sugar and vanilla to taste. Beat the eggs well while the milk is being heated. Use vanilla pods to flavour—they are better than the essence, which is alcoholic; split a piece of the pod 3 or 4 inches long, and let it soak in the milk for 1 hour before it is set over the fire, so as to extract the flavour from the vanilla. Sweeten the milk and let it come nearly to boiling-point. Carefully stir the milk into the beaten eggs, adding only a little at a time, so as not to curdle the eggs. When all is mixed, pour the custard into a jug, which should be placed in a saucepanful of boiling water. Keep stirring the custard with a wooden spoon, and as soon as the custard begins to coat the spoon remove the saucepan from the fire, and continue stirring the custard until it is well thickened. In doing as here directed there is no risk of the custard curdling, for directly the water ceases to boil it cannot curdle the custard, although it is hot enough to finish thickening it. If the milk is nearly boiling when mixed with the eggs, the custard will only take from 5 to 10 minutes to finish. When the custard is done place the jug in which it was made in a bowl of cold water, stir it often while cooling to prevent a skin forming on the top. Remove the vanilla pod and pour the custard into glasses. Should the custard be required very thick, 8 eggs should be used, or the milk can first be thickened with a dessertspoonful of

Allinson cornflour before mixing it with the 6 eggs. This is an excellent plan; it saves eggs, and the custard tastes just as rich as if more eggs were used. Serve in custard glasses, or in a glass dish.

CUSTARD (ALLINSON).

1 pint of milk or cream, 2 oz. of lump sugar and 1 packet of Allinson custard powder. Put the contents of the packet into a basin and mix to a smooth, thin paste with about 2 tablespoonfuls of the milk; boil the remainder of milk with the sugar, and when quite boiling pour quickly into the basin, stirring thoroughly; stir occasionally until quite cold, then pour into custard glasses and grate a little nutmeg on the top, or put in a glass dish and serve with stewed or tinned fruits, or the custard can be used with Christmas or plum pudding instead of sauce.

When the custard has been standing over night, it should be well stirred before using.

CUSTARD IN PASTRY OR KENTISH PUDDING PIE.

Line a pie-dish with puff paste, prick well with a fork and bake carefully, then fill the case with a custard made as follows. Mix 1 dessertspoonful of flour with the contents of a packet of Allinson custard powder, out of a pint of milk take 8 tablespoonfuls and mix well with the flour, custard powder, &c., boil the remainder of milk with sugar to taste and 1 oz. of butter and when quite boiling pour on to the custard powder, stir quickly for a minute, then pour into the pastry case, grate a little nutmeg on the top and bake till of a golden brown; serve either hot or cold.

FRUMENTY.

1 quart of milk, ½ pint of ready boiled wheat (boiled in water), ¼ lb. of sultanas and currants mixed, sugar to taste, 4 eggs, a stick of cinnamon. Mix the milk with the wheat (which should be fresh), the sugar and fruit, adding the cinnamon, and let all cook gently over a low fire, stirring frequently; when the mixture is nicely thickened remove it from the fire and let it cool; beat up the eggs and gradually mix them with the rest, taking great care not to curdle them. Stir the frumenty over the fire, but do not allow to boil. Serve hot or cold. The wheat should be fresh and soaked for 24 hours, and then cooked from 3 to 5 hours.

GOOSEBERRY CUSTARD.

Make some good puff paste and line a pie-dish with it, putting a double row round the edge. With ½ lb. of castor sugar stew 1 lb. of green gooseberries until the skins are tender, then rub them through a sieve. Scald 1 pint of milk, mix 1 tablespoonful of Allinson cornflour to a smooth paste with cold milk, add it to the milk when boiling, let it boil for 5 minutes, gently stirring it all the time, then turn it into a bowl and let it become cool. Add ¼ lb. of castor sugar, 2 oz. of butter melted and dropped in gradually whilst the mixture is beaten, then put in the well-beaten yolks of 6 eggs, add the mashed gooseberries in small quantities, and lastly the whites of the eggs whipped to a stiff froth; beat all together for a minute to mix well. Pour this into the lined pie-dish and bake 25 or 30 minutes; serve in the pie-dish. This can be made from any kind of acid fruit, and is as good cold as hot.

GOOSEBERRY FOOL.

Top and tail 1 pint of gooseberries, put into a lined saucepan with sugar to taste and half a small teacupful of water, stew gently until perfectly tender, rub through a sieve, and when quite cold add 1 pint of custard made with Allinson custard powder, which should have been allowed to become cold before being mixed with the fruit. Serve in a glass dish with sponge fingers.

N.B.—Apple fool is made in exactly the same way as above, substituting sharp apples for the gooseberries.

MACARONI CUSTARD.

4 oz. of Allinson macaroni, 3 eggs, 1 tablespoonful of sugar, 1 even dessertspoonful of Allinson cornflour, vanilla to taste. Boil the macaroni in 1 pint of milk, and add a little water it needed; when quite tender place it on a glass dish to cool; make a custard of the rest of the milk and the other ingredients; flavour it well with vanilla; when the custard is cool pour it over the macaroni, and serve with or without stewed fruit.

MACAROON CUSTARD.

½ lb. of macaroons, 1 quart of milk, 6 eggs, 1 dessertspoonful of Allinson cornflour, sugar and vanilla essence to taste. Boil the milk and stir into it the cornflour smoothed with a little of the milk; whip up the eggs, and carefully stir in the milk (which should have been allowed to go off the boil) without curdling it; add sugar and vanilla to taste, and stir the custard over the fire until it thickens, placing it in a jug into a saucepan of boiling water. Arrange the macaroons in a glass dish, and when the custard is cool enough not to crack the dish, pour it over them and sprinkle some ground almonds on the top. Serve cold.

ORANGE CUSTARD.

The juice of 6 oranges and of ½ a lemon, 6 eggs, 6 oz. of sugar, and 1 dessertspoonful of Allinson cornflour. Add enough water to the fruit juices to make 1-1/2 pints of liquid. Set this over the fire with the sugar; meanwhile smooth the cornflour with a little cold water, and thicken the liquid with it when boiling. Set aside the saucepan, (which should be an enamelled one) so as to cool the contents a little. Beat up the eggs, gradually stir into them the thickened liquid, and then proceed with the custard as in the previous recipe. This is a German sweet, and very delicious.

RASPBERRY CUSTARD.

1-1/2 pints of raspberries, ½ pint of red currants, 6 oz. of sugar, 7 eggs, 1 dessertspoonful of Allinson cornflour. Mix the fruit, and let it cook from 5 to 10 minutes with 1 pint of water; strain the juice well through a piece of muslin or a fine hair-sieve. There should be 1 quart of juice; if necessary add a little more water; return the juice to the saucepan, add the sugar and reheat the liquid; when it boils thicken it with the cornflour, then set it aside to cool. Beat up the eggs, add them carefully after the fruit juice has somewhat cooled; stir the custard over the fire until it thickens, but do not allow it to boil, as the eggs would curdle. Serve cold in custard glasses, or in a glass dish poured over macaroons or sponge cakes. You can make a fruit custard in this way, with strawberries, cherries, red currants, or any juicy summer fruit.

STRAWBERRY CUSTARD.

Remove the stalks from 1 lb. of fresh strawberries, place them in a glass dish and scatter over 2 tablespoonfuls of pounded sugar; prepare 1 pint of custard with Allinson custard powder according to recipe given above, and while still hot pour carefully over the fruit, set aside to cool, and just before serving (which must not be until the custard has become quite cold) garnish the top with a few fine strawberries.

APPLE COOKERY

APPLES (BUTTERED).

1 lb. of apples, 2 oz. of butter, ground cinnamon and sugar to taste. Pare, core, and slice the apples; heat the butter in a frying-pan, when it boils turn in the apples and fry them until cooked; sprinkle with sugar and cinnamon, and serve on buttered toast.

APPLE CAKE

6 oz. each of Allinson fine wheatmeal and white flour, 4-1/2 oz. of butter, 1 egg, a little cold water, 1-1/2 lbs. of apples, 1 heaped-up teaspoonful of cinnamon, and 3 oz. of castor sugar. Rub the butter into the meal and flour, beat up the egg and add it, and as much cold water as is required to make a smooth paste; roll out the greater part of it ¼ inch thick, and line a flat buttered tin with it. Pare, core, and cut the apples into thin divisions, arrange them in close rows on the paste point down, leaving 1 inch of edge uncovered; sift the sugar and cinnamon over the apples; roll out thinly the rest of the paste, cover the apples with it, turn up the edges of the bottom crust over the edges of the top crust, make 2 incisions in the crust, and bake the cake until brown in a moderately hot oven; when cold sift castor sugar over it, slip the cake off the tin, cut into pieces, and serve.

APPLE CHARLOTTE.

2 lbs. of good cooking apples, 2 oz. of chopped almonds, 4 oz. of currants and sultanas mixed, 1 stick of cinnamon about 3 inches long, sugar

to taste, the juice of ½ a lemon, and Allinson bread and butter cut very thinly. Pare, core, and cut up the apples, and stew them with a teacupful of water and the cinnamon, until the apples have become a pulp; remove the cinnamon, and add sugar, lemon juice, the almonds, and the currants and sultanas, previously picked, washed, and dried; mix all well and allow the mixture to cool; butter a pie-dish and line it with thin slices of bread and butter, then place on it a layer of apple mixture, repeat the layers, finishing with slices of bread and butter; bake for ¾ hour in a moderate oven.

APPLES (DRYING).

Those who have apple-trees are often at a loss to know what to do with the windfalls. The apples come down on some days by the bushel, and it is impossible to use them all up for apple pie, puddings, or jelly. An excellent way to keep them for winter use is to dry them. It gives a little trouble, but one is well repaid for it, for the home-dried apples are superior in flavour to any bought apple-rings or pippins. Peel your apples, cut away the cores and all the worm-eaten parts—for nearly the whole of the windfalls are more or less worm-eaten. The good parts cut into thin pieces, spread them on large sheets of paper in the sun. In the evening (before the dew falls), they should be taken indoors and spread on tins (but with paper underneath), on the cool kitchen stove, and if the oven is only just warm, placed in the oven well spread out; of course they require frequent turning about, both in the sun and on the stove. Next day they may again be spread in the sun, and will probably be quite dry in the course of the day. Should the weather be rainy, the apples must be dried indoors only, and extra care must then be taken that they are neither scorched nor cooked on the stove. Whilst cooking is going on they will dry nicely on sheets of paper on the plate-rack. When the apples are quite dry, which is when the outside is not moist at all, fill them into brown paper bags and hang them up in an airy, dry place. The apples will be found delicious in flavour when stewed, and most acceptable when fresh fruit is scarce. I have dried several bushels of apples in this way every year.

APPLE DUMPLINGS.

Core as many apples as may be required. Fill the holes with a mixture of sugar and cinnamon; make a paste for a short crust, roll it out, and wrap each apple in it. Bake the dumplings about 30 or 40 minutes in the oven, or boil them the same time in plenty of water, placing the dumplings in the water when it boils fast. Serve with cream or sweet white sauce.

APPLE FOOL.

2 lbs. of apples, ½ lb. of dates, ¾ pint of milk, ¼ pint of cream, 6 cloves tied in muslin, and a little sugar. Pare, core, and cut up the apples, stone the dates, and gently stew the fruit with a teacupful of water and the cloves until quite tender; when sufficiently cooked, remove the cloves, and rub the fruit through a sieve; gradually mix in the milk, which should be boiling, then the cream; serve cold with sponge-cake fingers.

APPLE FRITTERS.

3 good juicy cooking apples, 3 eggs, 6 oz. of Allinson fine wheatmeal, ½ pint of milk, and sugar to taste. Pare and core the apples, and cut them into rounds ¼ inch thick; make a batter with the milk, meal, and the eggs well beaten, adding sugar to taste. Have a frying-pan ready on the fire with boiling oil, vege-

butter, or butter, dip the apple slices into the batter and fry the fritters until golden brown; drain them on blotting paper, and keep them hot in the oven until all are done.

APPLE JELLY.

1 pint of water to each 1 lb. of apples. Wash and cut up the apples, and boil them in the water until tender; then pour them into a jelly bag and let drain well; take 1 lb. of loaf sugar to each pint of juice, and the juice of 1 lemon to each quart of liquid. Boil the liquid, skimming carefully, until the jelly sets when cold if a drop is tried on a plate. It may take from 2 hours to 3 hours in boiling.

APPLE PANCAKES.

Make the batter as directed in the recipe for "Apple Fritters," peel 2 apples, and cut them in thin slices, mix them with the batter, add sugar and cinnamon to taste, a little lemon juice if liked, and fry the pancakes in the usual way.

APPLE PUDDING.

1-1/2 lbs. of apples, 1 teaspoonful of ground cinnamon, sugar to taste, ½ lb. of Allinson fine wheatmeal, and 2-1/2 oz. of butter or vege-butter. Pare, core, and cut up the apples; make a paste of the meal, butter and a little cold water; roll the paste out, line a pudding basin with the greater part of it, put in the apples, and sprinkle over them the cinnamon and 4 oz. of sugar—a little more should the apples be very sour; cover the apples with the rest of the paste, and press the edges together round the sides; tie a cloth over the basin and boil the pudding for 2-1/2 to 3 hours in a saucepan with boiling water.

APPLE PUDDING (Nottingham).

6 baking apples, 2 oz. of sugar, 1 heaped up teaspoonful of ground cinnamon, ¾ pint of milk, 3 eggs, 6 oz. of Allinson wholemeal, and 1 oz. of butter. Core the apples, mix the sugar and cinnamon, and fill the hole where the core was with it; put the apples into a buttered pie-dish; make a batter of the milk, eggs, and meal, melt the butter and mix it into the batter; pour it over the apples, and bake the pudding for 2 hours in a moderate oven.

APPLE SAGO.

5 oz. of sago, 1-1/2 lbs. of apples, the juice of a lemon, a teaspoonful of ground cinnamon, and sugar to taste. Wash the sago and cook it in 1-1/2 pints of water, to which the cinnamon is added; meanwhile have the apples ready, pared, cored, and cut up; cook them in very little water, just enough to keep the apples from burning; when they are quite soft rub them through a sieve and mix them with the cooking sago, adding sugar and lemon juice; let all cook gently for a few minutes or until the sago is quite soft; put the mixture into a wetted mould, and turn out when cold.

APPLE SAUCE.

1 lb. of good cooking apples, sugar to taste. Pare, core, and cut in pieces the apples, cook them in a few spoonfuls of water to prevent them burning; when quite soft rub the apple through a sieve, and sweeten the sauce to taste. Rubbing the sauce through a sieve ensures the sauce being free from pieces should the apple not pulp evenly.

APPLE TART (OPEN).

2 lbs. of apples, 1 cupful of currants and sultanas, 2 oz. of chopped almonds, sugar to taste, 1 teaspoonful of ground cinnamon or the rind of ½ lemon (which latter should be

removed after cooking with the apples), 12 oz. or Allinson fine wheatmeal, and 4-1/2 oz. of butter. Pare, core, and cut up the apples; stew them in very little water, only just enough to keep from burning; when nearly done add the currants, sultanas, almonds, cinnamon, and sugar; let all simmer together until the apples have become a pulp; let the fruit cool; make a paste of the meal, butter, and a little water; roll it out and line a round, flat dish with it, and brush the paste over with white of eggs; turn the apple mixture on the paste; cut the rest of the paste into strips 3/8 of an inch wide, and lay them over the apples in diamond shape, each 1 inch from the other, so as to make a kind of trellis arrangement of the pastry. If enough paste is left, lay a thin strip right round the dish to finish off the edge, mark it nicely with a fork or spoon, and bake the tart for ¾ hour. Serve with white sauce or custard.

APPLES (RICE)

2 lbs. of apples, ½ lb. of rice, the rind of ½ lemon (or a piece of stick cinnamon if preferred), 4 oz. of sultanas, sugar to taste, 1 oz. of butter, and, if the apples are not sour, the juice of a lemon. Boil the rice in 3 pints of water with the lemon rind, then add the apples, pared, cored, and sliced, the sultanas, butter, lemon juice, and sugar; let all simmer gently for ½ hour, or until quite tender; if too dry add a little more water; remove the lemon rind before serving.

EVE PUDDING.

½ lb. each of apples and breadcrumbs, and ½ lb. of currants and sultanas mixed, 5 eggs well beaten, sugar to taste, the grated rind and juice of 1 lemon, and 2 oz. of butter. Peel, core, and chop small the apples, mix them with the breadcrumbs, sugar, currants, and sultanas (washed and picked), the lemon juice and rind, and the butter, previously melted; whip up the eggs and mix them well with the other ingredients; turn the mixture into a buttered mould, tie with a cloth, and steam the pudding for 3 hours.

BREAD AND CAKES

THE ADVANTAGES OF WHOLEMEAL BREAD.

People are now concerning themselves about the foods they eat, and inquiring into their properties, composition, and suitability. One food that is now receiving a good deal of attention is bread, and we ought to be sure that this is of the best kind, for as a nation we eat daily a pound of it per head. We consume more of this article of food than of any other, and this is as it ought to be, for bread is the staff of life, and many of the other things we eat are garnishings. It is said we cannot live on bread alone, but this is untrue if the loaf is a proper one; at one time our prisoners were fed on it alone, and the peasantry of many countries live on very little else.

Not many years ago books treating of food and nutrition always gave milk as the standard food, and so it is for calves and babies. Nowadays we use a grain food as the standard, and of all grains wheat is the one which is nearest perfection, or which supplies to the body those elements that it requires, and in best proportions. A perfect food must contain carbonaceous, nitrogenous, and mineral matter in definite quantities; there must be from four to six parts of carbonaceous or heat and force-forming matter to one of nitrogen, and from two to four per cent. of mineral matter; also a certain bulk of innutritious matter for exciting secretion, for separating the particles of food so that the various gastric and intestinal juices may penetrate and dissolve out all the nutriment, and for carrying off the excess of the biliary and other intestinal secretions with the fæces.

A grain of wheat consists of an outer hard covering or skin, a layer of nitrogenous matter directly under this, and an inner kernel of almost pure starch. The average composition of wheat is this:—

Nitrogen	12
Carbon	72
Mineral Matter	4
Water	12
	100

From this analysis we observe that the nitrogenous matter is to the carbonaceous in the proportion of one-sixth, which is the composition of a perfect food. Besides taking part in this composition, the bran, being in a great measure insoluble, passes in bulk through the bowels, assisting daily laxation—a most important consideration. If wheat is such a perfect food, it must follow that wholemeal bread must be best for our daily use. That such is the case, evidence on every side shows; those who eat it are healthier, stronger, and more cheerful than those who do not, all other things being equal. Wholemeal bread comes nearer the standard of a perfect food than does the wheaten grain, as in fermentation some of the starch is destroyed, and thus the proportion of nitrogen is slightly increased.

The next question is, how shall we prepare the grain so as to make the best bread from it? This is done by grinding the grain as finely as possible with stones, and then using the resulting flour for bread-making. The grain should be first cleaned and brushed, and passed over a magnet to cleanse it from any bits of steel or iron it may have acquired from the various processes it goes through, and then finely ground. To ensure fine grinding, it is always advisable to kiln-dry it first. When ground, nothing must be taken from it, nor must anything be added to the flour, and from this bread should be made. Baking powder, soda, and tartaric acid, or soda and hydrochloric acid, or ammonia and hydrochloric acid, or other chemical agents, must never be used for raising bread, as these substances are injurious, and affect the human system for harm. The only ferment that should be used is yeast; of this the French variety is best. If brewer's yeast is used it must be first well washed, otherwise it gives a bitter flavour to the loaf. A small quantity of salt may be used, but not much, otherwise it adds an injurious agent to the bread.

BARLEY BANNOCKS.

Put ½ pint of milk into a saucepan allow it to boil; then sprinkle in barley meal, stirring it constantly to prevent lumps till the mixture is quite thick and almost unstirrable. Turn the mass out on a meal-besprinkled board and leave to cool. When cool enough to knead, work it quite stiff with dry meal, take a portion off, roll it as thin as a wafer, and bake it on a hot girdle; when done on one side, turn and cook on the other. The girdle is to be swept clean after each bannock. Eat hot or cold with butter.

BUN LOAF.

1 lb. Allinson wholemeal flour, ½ lb. butter, ½ lb. brown sugar, ¼ lb. currants, ¼ lb. raisins, ¼ lb. candied peel, 4 eggs, ½ teacupful of milk. Mix the flour, sugar, currants, raisins, candied peel (cut in thin strips), the butter and eggs well together; mix with the milk; pour into a buttered tin, and bake in a moderate oven for 2 hours.

BUNS (1).

1 lb. flour, ¼ lb. sugar, 4 oz. currants, 2 oz. butter, or vege-butter, 1 teacupful of milk, 1 oz. French yeast, 2 eggs, a little salt. Mix the flour, sugar, salt, and currants in a basin, warm the butter and milk slightly, mix it smoothly with the yeast, then add the eggs well beaten; pour this on the flour, stirring well together till it is all moistened; when thoroughly mixed, set it to rise by the fire for ½ hour; make into buns, set to rise by the fire for 10 minutes, brush the tops over with egg, and bake from 10 to 15 minutes.

BUNS (2).

½ pint water, ½ pint milk, 1 oz. yeast, 1 oz. sugar, 6 oz. Allinson's wholemeal, 1 egg (not necessary). Warm water and milk to 105 degrees, dissolve sugar and yeast in it and stir in the meal, leave well covered up in a warm place for 45 minutes. Then have ready 1 ¾ lbs. Allinson's wholemeal, ¼ lb. vege-butter, 5 oz. sugar, ½ lb. currants, pinch of salt. Melt down vege-butter to oil, make bay of meal, sprinkle currants round, stir the sugar and salt with the ferment till dissolved, then mix in the melted butter and make up into a dough with the meal and currants. Keep in warm place for 45 minutes, then knock gas out of dough and leave ½ hour more; shape buns, place on warm greased tin, prove 15 minutes and bake in moderately warm oven for 20 minutes.

BUNS (PLAIN).

1 lb. flour, 6 oz. butter, or vege-butter, ¼ lb. sugar, 1 egg, ¼ pint milk, 15 drops essence of lemon. Warm the butter without oiling it, beat it with a wooden spoon, stir the flour in gradually with the sugar, and mix the ingredients well together; make the milk lukewarm, beat up with it the egg and lemon

and stir to the flour; beat the dough well for 10 minutes, divide into 24 pieces, put into patty pans, and bake in a brisk oven for from 20 to 30 minutes.

BUTTER BISCUITS.

½ lb. butter, 2 lbs. fine wholemeal flour, ½ pint milk. Dissolve the butter in the milk, which should be warmed, then stir in the meal and make into a stiff, smooth paste, roll it out very thin, stamp it into biscuits, prick them out with a fork, and bake on tins in a quick oven for 10 minutes.

BUTTERMILK CAKE.

2 lbs. Allinson wholemeal flour, 2 lbs. currants, ½ lb. sugar, 12 oz. butter, 2 oz. candied lemon peel, 1 pint buttermilk. Beat the butter to a cream, add the sugar, then the meal, fruit, and milk, mix thoroughly; butter a cake tin, pour in the mixture, and bake in a slow oven for 3 ½ hours.

BUTTERMILK CAKES.

2 lbs. wholemeal flour, 1 pint buttermilk, 1 teaspoonful salt. Mix the meal well with the salt, add the buttermilk and pour on the flour; beat well together, roll it out, cut into cakes, and bake for from 15 to 20 minutes in a quick oven.

CHOCOLATE BISCUITS.

2 oz. of powdered chocolate, 2 oz. of white sugar, 2 whites of eggs beaten to a stiff froth. Mix all together, and drop in biscuits on white or wafer paper. Bake 16 minutes in a moderate oven.

CHOCOLATE CAKE (1).

½ lb. of fine wheatmeal, ¼ lb. of butter, 5 eggs, ½ lb. of castor sugar, 1-1/2 oz. of Allinson cocoa, 1 dessertspoonful of vanilla essence. Proceed as in recipe of "Madeira Cake," adding the cocoa and flavouring with vanilla.

CHOCOLATE CAKE (2).

Work 4 oz. of butter to a cream, add a ¼ lb. of castor sugar, 3 eggs, and a little milk. Mix together ½ lb. of Allinson fine wheatmeal, a heaped tablespoonful of cocoa. Add to the butter mixture, and bake on a shallow tin or plate in a quick oven. The cake can be iced when done, and cut, when cold, into diamond-shaped pieces or triangles.

CHOCOLATE MACAROONS.

½ lb. of ground sweet almonds, 1 oz. of cocoa, 1 dessertspoonful of vanilla essence, ½ lb. of castor sugar, the white of 4 eggs. Whip the white of the eggs to a stiff froth, add the sugar, cocoa, vanilla, and almond meal, and proceed as in the previous recipe.

CINNAMON MADEIRA CAKE.

½ lb. of fine wheatmeal, ¼ lb. of butter, ½ lb. of sugar, ¼ lb. of currants and sultanas mixed (washed and picked) 5 eggs, 1 dessertspoonful of ground cinnamon. Proceed as in recipe for "Madeira Cake," adding the fruit, and cinnamon as flavouring.

COCOANUT BISCUITS.

2 breakfastcupfuls of wheatmeal, 2 teacupfuls of grated cocoanut, 3 dessertspoonfuls of sugar, 3 tablespoonfuls of orange water, 2 oz. of butter, a little milk. Mix the ingredients, adding a little milk to moisten the paste, mix it well, roll the paste out ¼ in. thick, cut out with

a biscuit cutter. Prick the biscuits, and bake them in a moderate oven a pale brown.

COCOANUT DROPS.

½ lb. of desiccated cocoanut, ½ lb. of castor sugar, the whites of 3 eggs. Beat the whites of the eggs to a stiff froth, add the sugar, then the cocoanut. Place little lumps of the mixture on the rice wafer paper, as in recipe for "Macaroons," and bake in a fairly hot oven.

COCOANUT ROCK CAKES.

1 lb. of fine wholemeal flour, 6 oz. of desiccated cocoanut, 3 oz. of butter, 3 eggs, a little cold milk, 6 oz. castor sugar. Rub the butter into the meal, add the sugar, cocoanut, and the well-beaten eggs. Mix, and add only just enough milk to make the mixture keep together. Put small lumps on a floured baking tin, and bake in a quick oven.

CORNFLOUR CAKE.

½ lb. of cornflour, 4 eggs, 6 oz. butter, same of castor sugar; separate the yolks of eggs from the whites and beat separately for a ¼ of an hour, cream the butter and sugar, mix with the yolks, then the whites, and lastly the flour, and whisk all together for 25 minutes, and bake for 1 hour in a moderately hot oven.

CRACKERS.

1 cupful butter, 1 teaspoonful salt, 2 quarts Allinson wholemeal flour. Rub thoroughly together with the hand, and wet up with cold water; beat well, and beat in meal to make brittle and hard; then pinch off pieces and roll out each cracker by itself, if you wish them to resemble baker's crackers.

CRISP OATMEAL CAKES.

1 lb. of oatmeal, 2 oz. of butter or oil (1 tablespoonful of oil is 1 oz.), 1 gill of cold milk. Make a dough of the butter, meal, and milk; shake meal plentifully on the board, turn the dough on to it, and having sprinkled this too with meal, work it a little with the backs of your fingers. Roll the dough out to the thickness of a crown piece, cut it in shapes, put the cakes on a hot stove, and when they are a little brown on the underside, take them off and place them on a hanger in front of the fire in order to brown the upper side; when this is done they are ready for use.

DYSPEPTICS' BREAD.

9 oz. of Allinson wholemeal, 1 egg, a scant ½ pint of milk and water. Separate the yolk from the white of the egg. Beat up the yolk with the milk and water, and mix this with the meal into a thick batter; whip up the white of the egg stiff, and mix it well into the batter. Grease and heat a bread tin, turn the mixture into it, and bake the loaf for 1-1/2 hours in a hot oven. This is very delicious bread, very light and digestible.

DOUGHNUTS.

1-1/2 lbs. of wheatmeal, ¼ oz. yeast, 1 egg, 1 teaspoonful of cinnamon, 3 tablespoonfuls of sugar, enough lukewarm milk to moisten the dough, some jam and marmalade. Dissolve the yeast in a little warm milk, mix all the ingredients, adding the dissolved yeast and enough milk to make the dough sufficiently moist to handle. Let it rise 1-1/2 hours in front of the stove. When risen roll it out ½ in. thick, cut out round pieces, place a little jam or marmalade in the middle, close up the dough, forming the dough nuts, and cook them in boiling oil or vege-butter until brown and thoroughly done. Eat warm.

GINGER SPONGE CAKE (a nice Cake for Children who do not like Gingerbread).

3 breakfast cups of Allinson wholemeal flour, 1 breakfast cup of sugar, 3 eggs, 6 oz. of butter or vege-butter, 2 heaped teaspoonfuls of ground ginger, 1 saltspoonful of salt, ½ gill milk. Beat the butter, sugar, and eggs to a cream, mix all the dry ingredients together; add gradually to the butter, &c., lastly the milk. Put into a well-greased tin, bake about 20 minutes in a quick oven. When cold cut into finger lengths or squares.

ICING FOR CAKES.

To 8 oz. of sugar take 2 whites of eggs, well beaten, and 1 tablespoonful of orange-or rosewater. Whisk the ingredients thoroughly, and when the cake is cold cover it with the mixture. Set the cake in the oven to harden, but do not let it remain long enough to discolour.

JUMBLES.

1 lb. of wheatmeal, 1 lb. of castor sugar, ½ pint of milk, ¼ lb. of butter, 1 lb. ground almonds. Cream the butter, add the other ingredients, and moisten with a little rosewater. Roll out and cut the jumbles into any shape desired. Bake in a gentle oven.

LEMON CAKES.

½ lb. of castor sugar, ½ lb. of wheatmeal, sifted fine, the grated rind of a lemon, 2 oz. of butter, and 2 well-beaten eggs. Rub the butter into the meal, and mix all the ingredients well together; roll the mixture out thin, lay it on a tin, and when baked cut into diamond squares.

LIGHT CAKE.

2 lbs. of brown breadcrumbs, ½ lb. of sultanas, 3 eggs, yolks and whites beaten separately; 2 oz. of butter, as much milk as required to moisten ¼ lb. of sugar. Rub the butter into the breadcrumbs, add the fruit, sugar, yolks, and lukewarm milk. At the last add the whites beaten to a stiff froth. Put the mixture in a well-greased tin, and bake 1 hour in a moderate oven.

LUNCH CAKE.

A good lunch cake may be made by rubbing 6 oz. of butter into 1-1/4 lbs. of Allinson wholemeal flour, 6 oz. of sugar. Beat up the yolks of 4 eggs with a teacupful of milk, and work into the flour so as to make a stiff batter. Add 2 oz. of mixed peel cut small, and ½ lb. of mixed sultanas. Lastly, add the beaten white of the eggs, whisk well, and pour the mixture into a greased cake tin. Bake for 1-1/2 to 2 hours.

MACAROON.

½ lb. of ground sweet almonds, 1 oz. of ground bitter almonds, a few sliced almonds, the whites of 4 eggs, and ½ lb. of castor sugar. Whip the whites of the eggs to a stiff froth, add the sugar, then the almond meal, and mix all well; if the mixture seems very stiff add one or two teaspoonfuls of water. Lay sheets of kitchen paper on tins, over this sheets of rice wafers (or, as it is also called, "wafer paper"), which can be obtained from confectioners and large stores; drop little lumps of the mixture on the wafers, allowing room for the spreading of the macaroons, place a couple of pieces of sliced almond on each, and bake them in a quick oven until they are set and don't feel wet to the touch. If the macaroons brown too much, place a sheet of paper lightly over them.

MADEIRA CAKE.

½ lb. of fine wheatmeal, ½ lb. of castor sugar, ½ lb. of butter, 5 eggs, flavouring to taste. Beat the butter to a cream, add the sugar, then the eggs well beaten, the meal and the flavouring. Line a cake tin with buttered paper, and bake the cake in a moderate oven from 1 to 1-1/2 hours.

OATMEAL BANNOCKS.

Cold porridge, Allinson fine wheatmeal. Stir sufficient of the meal into any cold porridge that may be left over to form a dough just firm enough to roll out. Well grease and sprinkle with flour some baking sheets, roll the dough to the thickness of ½ an inch, cut into triangular shapes, and bake until brown on both sides. Butter and serve hot.

OATMEAL FINGER-ROLLS.

Use equal parts of medium oatmeal and Allinson fine wheatmeal, and add a good ½ pint of milk and water to 1 pound of the mixed meal. Knead into a dough, make it into finger-rolls about 3 inches long, and bake them in a quick oven from 30 to 40 minutes.

ORANGE CAKES.

6 oz. of Allinson wholemeal flour, 3 oz. butter, 4 oz. sugar, grate in the rind of 1 small orange, and mix all well together. Beat 1 egg, and stir in with the juice of the orange and sufficient buttermilk to make a smooth, thick batter. Half fill small greased tins with this mixture, and bake 15 minutes in a moderate oven.

PLAIN CAKE.

2-1/2 lbs. meal, 1 breakfastcupful sultanas, 1 oz. ground bitter almonds, 3 oz. chopped sweet almonds, 2 eggs, 3 oz. butter or ½ teacupful of oil, 6 oz. sugar and 1 teaspoonful cinnamon, ¼ oz. yeast, milk to moisten the cake. Dissolve the yeast in a cup of warm water, 100 degrees Fahrenheit in winter, 85 degrees in summer; make a batter of the yeast and water, with two spoonfuls of the meal, and stand it on a cool place of the stove to rise; do not let it get hot, as this will spoil the yeast. Meanwhile prepare the fruit and almonds, mix the meal, fruit, butter (or oil), sugar, cinnamon and eggs; then add the yeast and as much lukewarm milk as is required to moisten the cake. The dough should be fairly firm and wet. Let the dough rise in front of the fire. Fill into greased cake tins and bake for 1-1/2 hours.

POTATO FLOUR CAKES.

A ¼ lb. of potato flour, the same quantity of very fine wheatmeal (sift the latter through a sieve if not very fine), 4 oz. of castor sugar, 4 oz. of butter, the juice of ½ a lemon, 1 dessertspoonful of ground bitter almonds, and 1 egg. Cream the butter, which is done by beating the butter round the sides of the pan with a wooden spoon until it is quite creamy, add the egg well beaten, the lemon juice, then the sugar, meal, potato flour, and bitter almonds. Beat the mixture from 20 minutes to ½ an hour, then drop small lumps of it on floured tins, and bake the little cakes from 10 to 15 minutes.

QUEEN'S SPONGE CAKE.

¼ lb. cornflour, ¼ lb. wheatmeal, ½ lb. sifted sugar, 10 eggs, rind and juice of a lemon, some vanilla. Separate the yolks of the eggs from the whites; stir the yolks well, then sift in gradually, stirring all the time, the sugar and cornflour; add the lemon juice and rind; beat the whites of the eggs to a firm froth, mix it well with the rest; place the mixture in one or more greased cake tins and bake at once in a quick oven.

RICE CAKES (1).

1 lb. of ground rice, ¼ lb. of castor sugar, 6 eggs, 2 oz. of sweet and bitter ground almonds mixed. Mix the almonds with the ground rice, adding the sugar, and the eggs, well beaten; beat all together and bake the cake in a buttered mould, in a moderately hot oven.

RICE CAKES (2).

4 eggs, ½ lb. sugar, 6 oz. ground rice, lemon or almond flavouring. Beat the eggs a little, add the sugar and flour, and beat well; pour into a tin mould, greased and warmed, only half filling it, and bake in a moderate oven 1 hour.

RICE AND WHEAT BREAD.

Simmer 1 lb. of rice in 2 quarts of water until quite soft. Let it cool sufficiently to handle, and mix it thoroughly with 4 lbs. of wheatmeal; work in also ½ oz. of yeast dissolved in a very little lukewarm water or milk. Add a teaspoonful of salt. Knead well and set to rise before the fire 1-1/2 hours. Bake in a good hot oven.

ROCK SEED CAKES.

1 lb. of wholemeal, 4 oz. of sugar, 4 oz. of butter, 1 oz. of ground carraway seeds, about ¾ of a cupful of milk, and 3 eggs. Rub the butter into the meal, add sugar, seeds, the eggs well beaten, and the milk. Place the mixture in lumps on floured tins, and bake the cakes for half an hour in a hot oven.

SALLY LUNN.

¾ of lb. of Allinson wholemeal flour, 2 oz. salt butter, 1 egg, 1-1/2 gills of milk, ¼ an ounce of German yeast. Warm the milk and butter in a pan together, rub the yeast smooth with ½ a teaspoonful of sugar, add the milk and butter. Stir this mixture gradually into the flour, add the egg slightly beaten, mix till quite smooth. Divide into two, put into well-greased tins, set these in a warm place for 1 hour to rise. Put into a quick oven, and bake about 15 minutes.

SEED CAKE (1).

½ lb. fine wholemeal flour, 6 oz. butter, 6 oz. castor sugar, 2 eggs, ¼ oz. carraway seeds. Beat the butter and sugar to a cream, add the eggs well beaten, and dredge in the flour, add a little cold water it too dry. Bake for ½ an hour.

SEED CAKE (2).

1-1/2 lbs. of wholemeal, ½ lb. of butter, ¾ lb. of castor sugar, 1 oz. of ground carraway seeds, the yolks of 10 eggs, and the whites of 5 beaten to a stiff froth. Cream the butter, mix all the ingredients well together, adding the whites of the eggs last; line one or more tins with buttered paper, turn the mixture into them, and bake the cake or cakes from 1 to 1-1/2 hours, according to the size of the cakes and the heat of the oven. If a bright knitting needle passed through the cake comes out clean, the cake is done.

SEED CAKE (3).

The same as "Madeira Cake," adding ½ oz. of carraway seeds, ground fine, as flavouring.

SEED CAKE (4).

2 lbs. of meal, 6 oz. of sugar, 1 oz. of seed (crushed), ¼ oz. of yeast, 4 eggs, 3 oz. of

butter, and a little milk. Rub the butter into the meal, add the sugar, seed, and eggs; dissolve the yeast in warm milk and add to it the other ingredients. Moisten the dough with sufficient warm milk not to make it stick to your pan. Let the dough rise 1-1/2 hours in a warm place, fill into greased cake tins and bake the cakes 1-1/2 to 2 hours.

SEED CAKE (5).

4 eggs, their weight in sugar, meal and butter, ½ oz. of seed. Rub the butter to cream, then stir in gradually the other ingredients, first the eggs well beaten, then the sugar, the seed, and last the flour. Put in a greased tin and bake 1 to 1-1/2 hours.

SEED CAKE (6).

4 eggs, their weight in sugar, ½ their weight in butter, twice their weight in meal, ½ oz. of seed, a little lukewarm milk. Cream the butter first, then add the yolks of eggs, the sugar, seed, and meal, and enough milk to moisten the mixture; lastly, add the whites of the eggs beaten to a froth, and bake at once in a fairly quick oven.

SLY CAKES.

1 lb. Allinson wholemeal flour, 8 oz. butter, 8 oz. currants, 2 oz. sugar, and 6 drops essence of lemon; mix the flour and sugar, and make it into a smooth paste with water, but do not make it very wet. Roll out 3 times, and spread in the butter as for pastry; roll it very thin, and cut into rounds or square cakes. Spread half of them very thickly with currants, press the others very gently on the top, so as to form a sandwich, and bake in a quick oven till a light brown.

SPONGE CAKE (1).

6 oz. fine wheatmeal, ½ lb. castor sugar, 4 eggs, any flavouring to taste. Beat up the eggs, sift in the sugar, then the flour, and bake the mixture in a well-greased cake tin in a moderate oven from 1 to 1-1/2 hours.

SPONGE CAKE (2).

4 eggs, the weight of 3 in fine wheatmeal, and the weight of 4 in castor sugar, any flavouring to taste. Beat the eggs, sift in the sugar and meal, stirring all the time, add the flavouring, and pour the mixture into one or two greased cake tins, only filling them half full. Bake in a moderate oven for about an hour, until a knitting needle comes out clean.

SPONGE CAKE ROLY-POLY.

3 eggs, the weight of 2 in fine wheatmeal, of 8 in castor sugar, some raspberry and currant jam. Mix the ingredients as directed in "Sponge Cake," line a large, square, flat baking tin with buttered paper, pour the mixture into it, and bake it in a fairly hot oven from 7 to 12 minutes, or until baked through. Have a sheet of white kitchen paper on the kitchen table, on which sprinkle some white sugar. Turn the cake out of the tin on to the paper, spread the cake with jam, and roll up. This should be done quickly, for if the cake is allowed to cool it will not roll.

UNFERMENTED BREAD.

This is as sweet and pure a bread as the finger-rolls, and keeps fresh for several days, as it has to be mixed fairly moist. 2 lbs. of Allinson wholemeal, 1-1/2 pints of milk and water; mix these to a thick paste, and put the mixture into some small greased bread tins.

Loaves the size of the twopenny loaves will want 1-1/2 hours in a hot oven.

UNFERMENTED FINGER-ROLLS.

These are bread in the simplest and purest form, and liked by most. 1 lb. of Allinson wholemeal, a good ½ pint of milk and water mixed; mix the meal and the milk and water into a dough, knead it a few minutes, then make the dough into finger-rolls on a floured pastry-board, rolling the finger-rolls about 3 inches long with the flat hand. Place them on a floured baking-tin, and bake them in a sharp oven from ½ an hour to 1 hour. The time will depend on the heat of the oven. In a very hot oven the rolls will be well baked in ½ an hour.

VICTORIA SANDWICH.

Proceed the same as in "Sponge Cake Roly-Poly," but bake the mixture in 2 round, flat tins; spread jam on one, and cover with the other cake.

WHOLEMEAL BREAD (FERMENTED).

This will be found useful where a large family has to be provided for, or where it is desirable to bake bread for several days. 7 lbs. of Allinson wholemeal, 2-1/2 pints of warm water (about 85° Faht.), 1 teaspoonful salt, ½ oz. of yeast; dissolve the yeast in the water, add the salt, put the meal into a pan, make a hole in the centre of the meal, pour in the water with the yeast and salt, and mix the whole into a dough. Allow it to stand, covered with a cloth, 1-1/2 hours in front of the fire, turning the pan sometimes, so that the dough may get warm evenly. Then knead the dough well through, and if necessary add a little more warm water. Make the dough into round loaves, or fill it into greased tins, and bake it for 1-1/2 hours. The oven should be fairly hot. To know whether the bread is done, a clean skewer or knife should be passed through a loaf. It it comes out clean the bread is done; if it sticks it not sufficiently baked. When it is desired to have a soft crust, the loaves may be baked under tins in the oven.

WHOLEMEAL CAKE.

1 lb. of wholemeal, 4 oz. of sugar, 1 teaspoonful of cinnamon, 1 breakfastcupful of currants and sultanas mixed, well-washed and picked over, 3 oz. of chopped sweet almonds, 1 dozen ground bitter almonds, 3 eggs, ¼ oz. of German yeast, ¼ lb. Vegebutter, and some warm milk. Rub the butter into the meal, add the fruit, cinnamon, almonds and sugar, and the eggs well beaten. Dissolve the yeast in a cupful of warm milk (not hot milk) add it to the other ingredients, and make all into a moist dough, adding as much more milk as is required to make the dough sufficiently moist for the spoon to beat all together. Cover the pan in which you mix the cake with a cloth, place it in front of the fire, and allow the dough to rise 1-1/2 hours, turning the pan round occasionally that the dough may be equally warm. Then fill the dough into one or several well-greased tins, and bake the cake or cakes from 1 to 1-1/2 hours (according to the size) in a hot oven. If the cake browns too soon, cover it over with a sheet of paper.

WHOLEMEAL GEMS.

Mix Allinson wholemeal flour with cold water into a batter, pouring this into greased and hot gem pans, and baking for ¾ of an hour. All bread should be left for a day or two to set before it is eaten, otherwise it is apt to lie heavy on the stomach and cause a feeling of weight and uncomfortableness.

WHOLEMEAL ROCK CAKES.

1 lb. of meal, 3 oz. of butter or vege-butter, ¼ lb. of sugar, a cupful of currants and sultanas mixed, 3 oz. of blanched almonds, chopped fine, 1 teaspoonful of cinnamon, or the grated rind of half a lemon, 3 eggs, and very little milk (about ¾ of a teacup). Rub the butter into the meal, add the fruit, almonds, sugar, and cinnamon, beat up the eggs with the milk, and mix the whole to a stiff paste. Flour 1 or 2 flat tins, place little lumps of the paste on them, and bake the cakes in a quick oven 25 to 35 minutes. Particular care must be taken that the paste should not be too moist, as in that case the cakes would run. Vege-butter is a vegetable butter, made from the oil which is extracted from cocoanuts and clarified. It can be obtained from some of the larger stores, also from several depôts of food specialities. It is much cheaper than butter, and being very rich, goes further.

MISCELLANEOUS

A DISH OF SNOW.

1 pint of thick apple sauce, sweetened and flavoured to taste (orange or rosewater is preferable), the whites of 3 eggs, beaten to a stiff froth. Mix both together, and serve.

CAULIFLOWER AU GRATIN.

A fair-sized cauliflower, 1 pint of milk, 1-1/2 oz. of dried Allinson breadcrumbs, 3 oz. of cheese, 1-1/2 oz. of butter, 1 heaped-up tablespoonful of Allinson wholemeal flour, a little nutmeg, and pepper and salt to taste. Boil the cauliflower until half cooked, cut it into pieces, and place them in a pie-dish. Boil the milk, adding the seasoning, ½ oz. of the butter, and ½ a saltspoonful of the nutmeg. Thicken with the wholemeal smoothed in a little cold milk or water. Stir in the cheese and pour the sauce over the cauliflower. Shake the breadcrumbs over the top, cut the rest of the butter in bits, and place them over the breadcrumbs. Bake for 20 minutes to ½ an hour, or until the cauliflower is soft.

COMPÔTE OF ORANGES AND APPLES.

6 oranges, 8 fine sweet apples, 1 oz. of ground sweet almonds, syrup as in "Orange Syrup." Peel the oranges and the apples, cut them across in thin slices, coring the apples and removing the pips from the oranges. Arrange the fruit into alternate circles in a glass dish, sprinkling the ground almonds between the layers. Pour over the whole the syrup. Serve when cold.

CRUST FOR MINCE PIES.

½ lb. of Allinson fine wheatmeal, ½ lb. of medium oatmeal, 6 oz. of butter or vege-butter, 1 cupful of cold water. Rub the butter into the flour, add the water, and mix all into a paste with a knife. Roll the paste out thin on a floured board, cut pieces out with a tumbler or biscuit cutter. Line with them small patty pans, and fill them with mincemeat; cover with paste, moisten the edges and press them together, and bake the mince pies in a quick oven; they will be done in 15 to 20 minutes.

GROUND RICE PANCAKES.

4 oz. of ground rice, 4 eggs, 1 pint of milk, jam, some sifted sugar, and powdered cinnamon; butter or oil for frying. Make a batter of the milk, eggs, and ground rice. Fry

thin pancakes of the mixture, sprinkle them with sugar and cinnamon, place a dessertspoonful of jam on each, fold up, sprinkle with a little more sugar; keep hot until all the pancakes are fried, and serve them very hot. When the pancakes are golden brown on one side, they should be slipped on a plate, turned back into the frying-pan, and fried brown on the other side.

MACARONI PANCAKES.

2 oz. of macaroni, ½ pint of milk, 3 eggs, 3 oz. of Allinson fine wheatmeal, sugar to taste, the grated rind of a lemon, butter, and 1 whole lemon. Throw the macaroni into boiling water and boil until quite soft; drain it and cut it into pieces 1 inch long. Make a batter of the eggs, meal, and milk, add the lemon rind, sugar, and the macaroni; fry pancakes of the mixture, using a small piece of butter not bigger than a walnut for each pancake. Sift sugar over the pancakes and serve them very hot with slices of lemon.

MINCEMEAT.

1 lb. of apples, 1 lb. of stoned raisins, 1 lb. of currants, 6 oz. of citron peel, 3 oz. of blanched almonds, ½ lb. butter. Chop the fruit up very finely, add the almonds cut up fine, oil the butter and mix well with the fruit. Turn the mincemeat into little jars, cover tightly, and keep in a dry and cool place.

MINCEMEAT (another).

1 lb. each of raisins, apples, and currants, ½ lb. of butter, ½ lb. of blanched and chopped almonds, ½ lb. of moist sugar, the juice of 4 lemons, and ½ lb. of mixed peel. Wash and pick the currants, wash and stone the raisins, peel, core, and quarter the apples, and cut up the mixed peel; then mince all up together,

and add the chopped almonds. Melt the butter, mix it thoroughly with the fruit, fill it into one or more jars, cover with paper, and tie down tightly.

ORANGE FLOWER PUFF.

½ pint of milk, 3 eggs, 4 ozs. of Allinson fine wheatmeal, and 2 tablespoonfuls of orange water, some butter or oil for frying. Make a batter of the milk, eggs (well beaten), and meal, add the orange water, and fry the batter in thin pancakes, powder with castor sugar, and serve.

ORANGE SYRUP.

The rind of 3 oranges, ½ pint of water, 4 oz. of sugar. Boil the ingredients until the syrup is clear, then strain it and pour over the fruit.

ORANGES IN SYRUP.

Peel 6 oranges, carefully removing all the white pith. Put the rinds of these into ½ pint of cold water; boil it gently for 10 minutes. Strain, and add to the water 6 oz, of loaf sugar. Boil it until it is a thick syrup, then drop into it the oranges, divided in sections, without breaking the skins. Only a few minutes cooking will be needed. The oranges are nicest served cold.

RASPBERRY FROTH.

The whites of 5 eggs, 3 tablespoonfuls of raspberry jam. Beat the whites of the eggs to a very stiff froth, then beat the jam up with it and serve at once in custard glasses. This recipe can be varied by using various kinds of jam.

RICE FRITTERS.

6 oz. of rice, 1 pint of milk, 8 oz. of sugar, 1 oz. of fresh butter, 6 oz. of apricot marmalade, 3 eggs. Let the rice swell in the milk with the butter and the sugar over a slow fire until it is tender—this will take about ½ of an hour; when the rice is done, strain off any milk there may be left. Mix in the apricot marmalade and the beaten eggs, stir it well over the fire until the eggs are set; then spread the mixture on a dish, about ½ an inch thick. When it is quite cold, cut it in long strips, dip them in a batter, and fry them a nice brown. Strew sifted sugar over them, and serve.

SNOWBALLS.

1-1/2 pints of milk, 4 eggs, sugar and vanilla to taste, and 1 tablespoonful of cornflour. Boil the milk with sugar and a piece of vanilla or with 1 dessertspoonful of vanilla essence. Smooth the cornflour with a little cold milk, and thicken the milk with it. Whip the whites of the eggs to a very stiff froth with 1 spoonful of castor sugar, and drop spoonfuls of the froth into the boiling milk. Allow to boil until the balls are well set, turning them over that both sides may get done. Lift the balls out with a slice, and place them in a glass dish. Beat up the yolks of the eggs, stir them carefully in the hot milk; let the custard cool, and pour it into the glass dish, but not over the snowballs, which should remain white.

SPONGE MOULD.

9 stale sponge cakes, some raspberry jam, 2 pints of milk, 8 oz. of Allinson cornflour, sugar to taste, a few drops of almond essence. Halve the sponge cakes, spread them with jam, arrange them in a buttered mould, and soak them with ½ pint of the milk boiling hot. Boil the rest of the milk and thicken it with the cornflour as for blancmange; flavour with the

essence and sugar; pour the mixture over the sponge cakes, and turn all out when cold.

STEWED PEARS AND VANILLA CREAM.

Get 1 tin of pears, open it, and turn the contents into an enamelled stewpan, add some sugar and liquid cochineal to colour the fruit, and let them stew a few minutes. Take out the pears carefully without breaking them, and let the syrup cook until it is thick. When the pears are cold lay them on a dish with the cores upwards, and with a spoon scoop out the core, and fill the space left with whipped cream flavoured with vanilla and sweetened; sprinkle them with finely shredded blanched almonds or pistachios, and pour the syrup round them.

SWISS CREAMS.

4 oz. of macaroons, a little raisin wine and 1 pint of custard, made with Allinson custard powder; lay the macaroons in a glass dish and pour over enough raisin wine to soak them, make the custard in the usual way, let it cool and then pour over the cakes; when quite cold garnish with pieces of bright coloured jelly.

TAPIOCA ICE.

1 teacupful of tapioca, ½ teacupful of sifted sugar, 1 tinned pineapple. Soak the tapioca over night in cold water; in the morning boil it in 1 quart of water until perfectly clear, and add the sugar and pineapple syrup. Chop up the pineapple and mix it with the boiling hot tapioca; turn the mixture into a wet mould. When cold turn it out and serve with cream and sugar.

TIPSY CAKE.

12 small sponge cakes, ½ lb. jam, 1 pint of custard made with Allinson custard powder.

Soak the sponge cakes in a little raisin wine, arrange them on a deep glass dish in four layers, spread a little jam on each layer and pour the custard round, decorate the top with candid cherries and almonds blanched and split.

A WEEK'S MENU

I have written the following menus to help those who are beginning vegetarianism. When first starting, most housewives do not know what to provide, and this is a source of anxiety. I occasionally meet some who have been vegetarians a long time, but confess that they do not know how to provide a nice meal. They usually eat the plainest foods, because they know of no tasty dishes. When visitors come, we like to provide tempting dishes for them, and show them that appetising meals can be prepared without the carcases of animals. I only give seven menus, that is, one for each day of the week; but our dishes can be so varied that we can have a different menu daily for weeks without any repetition. The recipes here written give a fair idea to start with. Instead of always using butter beans, or haricot beans, as directed in one of these menus, lentils or split peas can be substituted. I have not included macaroni cheese in these menus, because this dish is so generally known; it can be introduced into any vegetarian dinner. I have allowed three courses at the dinner, but they are really not necessary. I give them to make the menus more complete. A substantial soup and a pudding, or a savoury with vegetables and sauce and a pudding, are sufficient for a good meal. In our own household we rarely have more than two courses, and often only one course. This article will be of assistance to all those who are wishing to try a healthful and humane diet, and to those meat eaters who wish to provide tasty meals for vegetarian friends.

Anna P. Allinson.

4,   Spanish   Place,
Manchester   Square,
London, W.

MENU I.

TOMATO SOUP.

1 tin of tomatoes or 2 lbs. of fresh ones, 1 large Spanish onion or ½ lb. of smaller ones, 2 oz. of butter, pepper and salt to taste, 1 oz. of vermicelli and 2 bay leaves. Peel the onions and chop up roughly; brown them with the butter in the saucepan in which the soup is made. When the onion is browned, add the tomatoes (the fresh ones must be sliced) and 3 pints of water. Let all cook together for ½ an hour. Then drain the liquid through a sieve without rubbing anything through. Return the liquid to the saucepan, add the seasoning and the vermicelli; then allow the soup to cook until the vermicelli is soft, which will be in about 10 minutes. Sago, tapioca, or a little dried julienne may be used instead of the vermicelli.

VEGETABLE PIE.

½ lb. each of tomatoes, turnips, carrots, potatoes, 1 tablespoonful of sago, 1 teaspoonful of mixed herbs, 3 hard-boiled eggs, 2 oz. of butter, and pepper and salt to taste. Prepare the vegetables, scald and skin the tomatoes, cut them in pieces not bigger than a walnut, stew them in the butter and 1 pint of water until nearly tender, add the pepper and salt and the mixed herbs. When cooked, pour the vegetables into a pie-dish, sprinkle in the sago, add water to make gravy if necessary. Cut the hard-boiled eggs in quarters and place them on the top of the vegetables, cover with a crust made from Allinson wholemeal, and bake until it is brown.

SHORT CRUST.

10 oz. of Allinson wholemeal, 8 oz. of butter or vege-butter, 1 teacupful of cold water. Rub the butter into the meal, add the water, mixing the paste with a knife. Roll it out, cut strips to line the rim of the pie-dish, cover the vegetable with the crust, decorate it, and bake the pie as directed.

GOLDEN SYRUP PUDDING.

10 oz. of Allinson wholemeal, 3 eggs, 1 pint of milk, and ½ lb. of golden syrup. Grease a pudding basin, and pour the golden syrup into it; make a batter with the milk, meal, and eggs, and pour this into the pudding basin on the syrup, but do not stir the batter up with the syrup. Place a piece of buttered paper on the top of the batter, tie a cloth over the basin unless you have a basin with a fitting metal lid, and steam the pudding for 2 ½ hours in boiling water. Do not allow any water to boil into the pudding. Dip the basin with the pudding in it for 1 minute in cold water before turning it out, for then it comes out more easily.

MENU II.

CLEAR CELERY SOUP.

1 large head of celery or 2 small ones, 1 large Spanish onion, 2 oz. of butter, pepper and salt to taste, and 1 blade of mace. Chop the onion and fry it brown in the butter (or vege-butter)

in the saucepan in which the soup is to be made. When brown, add 4 pints of water, the celery washed and cut into pieces, the mace, the pepper and salt. Let all cook until the celery is quite soft, then drain the liquid from the vegetables. Return it to the saucepan, boil the soup up, and add 1 oz. of vermicelli, sago, or Italian paste; let the soup cook until this is quite soft, and serve with sippets of Allinson wholemeal toast.

BUTTER BEANS WITH PARSLEY SAUCE.

Pick the beans, wash them and steep them over night in boiling water, just covering them. Allow 2 or 3 oz. of beans for each person. In the morning let them cook gently in the water they are steeped in, with the addition of a little butter, until quite soft, which will be in about 2 hours. The beans should be cooked in only enough water to keep them from burning; therefore, when it boils away, add only just sufficient for absorption. The sauce is made thus: 1 pint of milk, 1 tablespoonful of Allinson wholemeal, a handful of finely chopped parsley, the juice of ½ a lemon, pepper and salt to taste. Boil the milk and thicken it with the meal, which should first be smoothed with a little cold milk, then last of all add the lemon juice, the seasoning, and the parsley. This dish should be eaten with potatoes and green vegetables.

GROUND RICE PUDDING.

1 quart of milk, 6 oz. of ground rice, 1 egg, and any kind of jam. Boil the milk, stir into it the ground rice previously smoothed with some of the cold milk. Let the mixture gook gently for 5 minutes, stir frequently, draw the saucepan to the side, and when it has ceased to boil add the egg well whipped, and mix well. Pour half of the mixture into a pie-dish, spread a layer of jam over it, then pour the rest of the

pudding mixture over the jam, and let it brown lightly in the oven.

MENU III.

CARROT SOUP.

4 good-sized carrots, 1 small head of celery, 1 fair sized onion, a turnip, 3 oz. of Allinson breadcrumbs, 1-1/2 oz. of butter, 1 blade of mace, pepper and salt to taste. Scrape and wash the vegetables, and cut them up small; set them over the fire with 3 pints of water, the butter, bread, and mace. Let all boil together until the vegetables are quite tender, and then rub them through a sieve. Return the mixture to the saucepan, season with pepper and salt, and if too thick add water to the soup, which should be as thick as cream. Boil the soup up, and serve.

CURRIED RICE AND TOMATOES.

½ lb. of Patna rice, 1 dessertspoonful of curry powder, salt to taste, and 1 oz. of butter. Wash the rice, put it over the fire in cold water, let it just boil up, then drain the water off. Mix 1 pint of cold water with the curry powder, put this over the fire with the rice, butter, and salt. Cover the rice with a piece of buttered paper and let it simmer gently until the water is absorbed. This will take about 20 minutes. Rice cooked this way will have all the grains separate. For the tomatoes proceed as follows: 1 lb. of tomatoes and a little butter, pepper, and salt. Wash the tomatoes and place them in a flat tin with a few spoonfuls of water; dust them with pepper and salt, and place little bits of butter on each tomato. Bake them from 15 to 20 minutes, according to the size of the tomatoes and the heat of the oven. Place the rice in the centre of a hot flat dish, put the tomatoes round it, pour the liquid over the rice, and serve.

APPLE CHARLOTTE.

2 lbs. of cooking apples, 1 teacupful of mixed currants and sultanas, 1 heaped-up teaspoonful of ground cinnamon, 2 oz. of blanched and chopped almonds, sugar to taste, Allinson wholemeal bread, and butter. Pare, core, and cut up the apples and set them to cook with a teacupful of water. Some apples require much more water than others. When they are soft add the fruit picked and washed, the cinnamon, and the almonds and sugar. Cut very thin slices of bread and butter, line a buttered pie-dish with them. Place a layer of apples over the buttered bread, and repeat the layers of bread and apples until the dish is full, finishing with a layer of bread and butter. Bake from ¾ of an hour to 1 hour.

MENU IV.

RICE SOUP.

3 oz. of rice, 4 oz. of grated cheese, 1 breakfastcupful of tomato juice, 1 oz. of butter, pepper and salt to taste. Boil the rice till tender in 2-1/2 pints of water, with the butter and seasoning. When quite soft, add the tomato juice and the cheese; stir until the soup boils and the cheese is dissolved, and serve. If too much of the water has boiled away, add a little more.

HOT-POT.

2 lbs. of potatoes, ¾ lb. of onions, 1 breakfastcupful of tinned tomatoes or ½ lb. of sliced fresh ones, 1 teaspoonful of mixed herbs, 1-1/2 oz. butter, pepper and salt to

taste. Those who do not like tomatoes can leave them out, and the dish will still be very savoury. The potatoes should be peeled, washed, and cut into thin slices, and the onions peeled and cut into thin slices. Arrange the vegetables and tomatoes in layers; dust a little pepper and salt between the layer, and finish with a layer of potatoes. Cut the butter into little bits, place them on the top of the potatoes, fill the dish with hot water, and bake the hot-pot for 2 hours or more in a hot oven. Add a little more hot water if necessary while baking to make up for what is lost in the cooking.

CABINET PUDDING.

4 slices of Allinson bread toasted, 1-1/4 pints of milk, 8 eggs, 1 oz. of butter, sugar to taste, 2 oz. of chopped almonds, 1 teacupful of mixed currants and sultanas and any kind of flavouring—cinammon, lemon, vanilla, or almond essence. Crush the toast in your hands, and soak it in the milk. Whip the eggs up, melt the butter, and add both to the soaked toast. Thoroughly mix all the various ingredients together. Butter a pie-dish and pour the pudding mixture into it; put a few bits of butter on the top, and bake the pudding for 1 hour in a moderately hot oven.

MENU V.

LEEK SOUP.

2 bunches of leeks, 1-1/2 pints of milk, 1 oz. of butter, 1 lb. of potatoes, pepper and salt to taste, and the juice of 1 lemon. Cut off the coarse part of the green ends of the leeks, and cut the leeks lengthways, so as to be able to brush out the grit. Wash the leeks well, and see no grit remains, then out them in short

pieces. Peel, wash, and cut up the potatoes, then cook both vegetables with 2 pints of water. When the vegetables are quite tender, rub them through a sieve. Return the mixture to the saucepan, add the butter, milk, and seasoning, and boil the soup up again. Before serving, add the Lemon juice; serve with sippets of toast or Allinson rusks.

MUSHROOM SAVOURY.

4 slices Allinson bread toast, 8 eggs, 1 pint of milk, 3 oz. of butter, 1 lb. of mushrooms, 1 small onion chopped fine, and pepper and salt to taste. Crush the toast with your hand and soak it in the milk; add the eggs well whipped. Peel, wash, and out up the mushrooms, and fry them and the onion in the butter. When they have cooked in the butter for 10 minutes add them to the other ingredients, and season with pepper and salt. Pour the mixture into a greased pie-dish and bake the savoury for 1 hour. Serve with green vegetables, potatoes, and tomato sauce.

CHOCOLATE MOULD.

1 quart of milk, 2 oz. of potato flour, 2 oz. of Allinson fine wheatmeal, 1 heaped-up tablespoonful of cocoa, 1 dessertspoonful of vanilla essence, and sugar to taste. Smooth the potato flour, wheatmeal, and cocoa with some of the milk. Add sugar to the rest of the milk, boil it up and thicken it with the smoothed ingredients. Let all simmer for 10 minutes, stir frequently, add the vanilla, and mix it well through. Pour the mixture into a wetted mould; turn out when cold, and serve plain or with cold white sauce.

MENU VI.

ARTICHOKE SOUP.

1 lb. each of artichokes and potatoes, 1 Spanish onion, 1 oz. of butter, 1 pint of milk, and pepper and salt to taste. Peel, wash, and cut into dice the artichokes, potatoes, and onion. Cook them until tender in 1 quart of water with the butter and seasoning. When the vegetables are tender rub them through a sieve. Return the liquid to the saucepan, add the milk and boil the soup up again. Add water it the soup is too thick. Serve with small dice of bread fried crisp in butter or vege-butter.

YORKSHIRE PUDDING.

4 eggs, ½ lb. of Allinson fine wheatmeal, 1 pint of milk, pepper and salt to taste, 1 oz. of butter. Thoroughly beat the eggs, make a batter of them with the flour and milk, and season it. Well butter a shallow tin, pour in the batter, and cut the rest of the butter in bits. Scatter them over the batter and bake it ¾ of an hour. Serve with vegetables, potatoes, and sauce. To use half each of Allinson breakfast oats and wheatmeal flour will be found very tasty.

BAKED CARAMEL CUSTARD.

1-1/2 pints of milk, 5 eggs, vanilla essence, 4 oz. of castor sugar for the caramel, and a little more sugar to sweeten the custard. Heat the milk, whip up the eggs, and carefully stir the hot milk into the beaten eggs; flavour with vanilla and sugar to taste. Meanwhile put the castor sugar into a small enamelled saucepan and stir it over a quick fire until it is quite melted and brown. Add about 2 tablespoonfuls of hot water to the caramel, stir thoroughly, and pour it into a tin mould or a cake tin. Let the caramel run all round the sides of the tin; pour in the custard, and bake it in a moderate oven, standing in a larger tin of boiling water, until the custard is set. Let it get cold, turn out, and serve. This is a very dainty sweet dish.

MENU VII.

POTATO SOUP.

2 lbs. of potatoes, ½ a stick of celery or the outer stalks of a head of celery, saving the heart for table use, 1 large Spanish onion, 1 pint of milk, 1 oz. of butter, a heaped-up tablespoonful of finely chopped Parsley, and pepper and salt to taste. Peel, wash, and cut in pieces the potatoes, peel and chop roughly the onion, prepare and cut in small pieces the celery. Cook the vegetables in 8 pints of water until they are quite soft. Rub them through a sieve, return the fluid mixture to the saucepan; add the milk, butter, and seasoning, and boil the soup up again; if too thick, add more water. Mix the parsley in the soup just before serving.

BREAD AND CHEESE SAVOURY.

½ lb. of Allinson bread, 3 oz. of grated cheese, 1 pint of milk, 3 eggs, pepper and salt to taste, a little nutmeg, and some butter. Cut the bread into slices and butter them; arrange in layers in a pie-dish, spreading some cheese between the layers, and dusting with pepper, salt, and a little nutmeg. Finish with a good sprinkling of cheese. Whip up the eggs, mix them with the milk, and pour the mixture over the bread and cheese in the pie-dish. Pour the custard back into the basin, and repeat the pouring over the contents of the pie-dish. If this is done two or three times, the top slices of bread and butter get soaked, and then bake better. This should also be done when a bread and butter pudding is made. Bake the savoury until brown, which it will be in about ¾ of an hour.

ORANGE MOULD.

The juice of 7 oranges and of 1 lemon, 6 oz. of sugar, 4 eggs, and 4 oz. of Allinson cornflour. Add enough water to the fruit juices to make 1 quart of liquid; put 1-1/2 pints of this over the fire with the sugar. With the rest smooth the cornflour and mix with it the eggs well beaten. When the liquid in the saucepan is near the boil, stir into it the mixture of egg and cornflour. Keep stirring the mixture over a gentle fire until it has cooked 5 minutes. Turn it into a wetted mould and allow to get cold, then turn out and serve.

A WEEK'S MENU

Nutritive Value and Chemical Composition of Various Fruits, Nuts, Grains, and Vegetables.

(Analysis of the *edible portion*.)

PROFESSOR ATWATER'S ANALYSIS.

	Proteid per cent.	Calories in one lb.
FRUIT—FRESH.		
Apples	.4	290
Apricots	1.1	270
Bananas	1.3	460
Blackberries	1.3	270
Cherries	1.0	365
Cranberries	.4	215
Currants	1.5	265
Figs	1.5	380
Grapes	1.3	450
Huckleberries	.6	345
Lemons	1.0	205
Musk-melons	.8	90
Nectarines	.6	305

Oranges	.8	240
Pears	.6	295
Persimmons	.8	630
Pineapple	.4	299
Plums	1.0	395
Pomegranates	1.5	460
Raspberries	1.0	255
Strawberries	1.0	180
Water-melons	.4	140
Whortleberries or Wimberries	.7	390

FRUIT—DRIED.

Apples	1.6	1350
Apricots	4.7	1290
Citron	.5	1525
Currants	2.4	1495
Dates	2.1	1615
Figs	4.3	1475
Grapes	2.8	1205
Pears	2.8	1635
Prunes	2.1	1400
Raisins	2.6	1605
Apricots (canned)	.9	340
Marmalade	.6	1585
Pears (canned)	.3	355
Pineapple "	.4	715

GREEN VEGETABLES

Artichoke	2.6	365
Asparagus	2.1	220
Beetroot	1.6	215
Cabbage	1.6	145
" (Curly)	4.1	215
" (Sprouts)	4.7	215
Carrots	1.1	210
Cauliflower	1.8	140
Celery	1.1	85
Corn (green)	3.1	470
Cucumber	.8	80
Dandelion	2.4	285
Egg Plant	1.2	130
Horseradish	1.4	230
Kohl Rabi	2.0	145
Leeks	1.2	150
Lettuce	1.2	90
Mushrooms	3.5	210
Olives (green)	1.1	1400
" (ripe)	1.7	1205
Onions	1.6	225
Parsnips	1.6	300
Potatoes (boiled)	2.5	440

" (chipped)	6.8	2675
" (raw)	2.2	385
" (sweet)	1.8	570
Pumpkins	1.3	135
Radishes	1.0	120
Rhubarb	.6	105
Spinach	2.1	110
Tomatoes	.9	105
Turnips	1.3	185

NUTS—SHELLED.

Acorns	8.1	2620
Almonds	21.0	3030
Beechnuts	21.9	3075
Brazil Nuts	17.0	3265
Butternuts	27.0	3165
Chestnuts (dried)	10.7	1875
" (fresh)	6.2	1125
Cocoanuts	5.7	2760
" desiccated	6.3	3125
Filberts (Hazels)	15.6	3290
Hickory	15.4	3345
Peanuts	25.8	2560
Peanut Butter	29.3	2825
Pecans	9.6	3435
Pine Kernels	34.0	2845
Pistachios	22.3	2995
Walnuts	18.0	3300
" Black }		
" Californian}	27.6	3105

GRAIN FOODS, ETC.

Barley Meal	10.5	1640
" Pearled	8.5	1650
Buckwheat Flour	6.4	1620
Corn Flour	7.1	1645
Corn Meal (granular)	9.2	1655
" Popped	10.7	1875
Hominy	8.3	1650
Oatmeal	16.1	1860
Oats (rolled)	16.7	1850
Rice	8.0	1630
Rye Flour	6.8	1630
" Meal	13.6	1665
Wheat Flaked	13.4	1690
" Flour, or Wholemeal	13.8	1675
" Germs	10.5	1695
" Gluten	14.2	1665
" Self-raising	10.2	1600
Macaroni	13.4	1665
" Spaghetti	12.1	1660

" Vermicelli	10.9	1625
Beans, small White	21.9	1675
" Lima or Butter	18.1	1625
Lentils	25.7	1620
Peas (dried)	24.6	1655
" (green)	7.0	465
Arrowroot	---	1815
Corn-starch	---	1675
Sago	9.0	1635
Tapioca	---	1650

CAKES.

Cake, Fruit	5.9	1760
" Gingerbread	5.8	1670
" Sponge	6.3	1795

BISCUITS.

All kinds, average	10.0	1800
Water	11.7	1835

BREAD.

Buns, Currant	6.7	1515
" Hot Cross	7.9	1275
Corn, Indian	7.9	1205
Cheap Bread	10.9	1255
Gluten	9.3	1160
Home-made Bread	9.1	1225
White Bread	9.2	1215
Whole-wheat Bread	9.7	1140
Rolls, Plain	9.7	1470
" Vienna	8.5	1300
" Water	9.0	1300
Rye	9.0	1180

VARIOUS.

Chocolate	12.9	2860
Cocoa	21.6	2320
Candy	---	1785
Honey	---	1520
Molasses (cane)	2.4	1290

INVALID COOKERY

BARLEY.

The plants *Hordeum Distichon* and *Hordeum Vulgare* supply most of the barley used in this country. Barley has been used as a food from time out of mind. We find frequent mention of it in the Bible, and in old Latin and Greek books. According to Pliny, an ancient Roman writer, the gladiators were called Hordearii, or "barley eaters," because they were fed on this grain whilst training. These Hordearii were like our pugilists, except that they often fought to the death. Barley has been used from very ancient days for making an intoxicating drink. In Nubia, the liquor made from barley was called Bouzah, from which we get our English word "booze," meaning an intoxicating drink. The first intoxicant drink made in this country was ale, and it was made from barley. Hops were not used for beer or ale in those days. Barley is a good food, and was the chief food of our peasantry until the beginning of the nineteenth century. Barley contains about 7 per cent. of sugar, and its flesh-forming matter is in the form of casin the same as is found in cheese. This casin is not elastic like the gluten of wheat, so that one cannot make a light bread from barley. Here is the chemical composition of barley meal:—

Flesh formers	7.5
Heat and force formers (carbon)[A]	76.0
Mineral matters	2.0
Water	14.5
100.0	

[A] There is 2.5 per cent. of fat in barley, and 7 per cent. of sugar.

From this analysis we can judge that barley contains all the constituents of a good food. In it we find casin and albumen for our muscles; starch, sugar, and fat to keep us warm and give force; and there is a fair percentage of mineral matter for our bones and teeth.

Allinson's prepared barley may be eaten as porridge or pudding (see directions), and is much more nourishing than rice pudding; it is also good for adding to broth or soup, and to vegetable stews, and is most useful for making gruel and barley water. Barley water contains a great deal of nourishment, more than beef tea, and it can be drunk as a change from tea, coffee, and cocoa. During illness I advise and use barley water and milk, mixed in equal parts, and find this mixture invaluable.

BARLEY FOR BABIES.

Put 1 teaspoonful of Allinson's barley into a breakfast cup; mix this perfectly smooth with cold milk and cold water in equal parts, until the cup is full. Pour into a saucepan and bring to the boil, stirring all the time to prevent it getting lumpy.

BARLEY GRUEL.

Mix 1 large tablespoonful of Allinson's barley with a little cold water, add to this 1 pint of boiling milk and water, boil together a few minutes, take from the fire, let cool, then eat. A little nutmeg gives a pleasant flavour.

BARLEY FOR INVALIDS AND ADULTS.

Use 3 teaspoonfuls of Allinson's barley to ½ pint of milk and water, and prepare as "Barley for Babies."

BARLEY JELLY.

Wash, then steep, 6 oz. of pearl barley for 6 hours, pour 31/2 pints of boiling water upon it, stew it quickly in a covered jar in a hot oven till perfectly soft and the water absorbed. When half done, add 6 oz. of sugar and a few drops of essence of lemon. 21/2 hours is the correct time for stewing the barley, and it is then a better colour than if longer in preparation. Pour it into a mould to set.

BARLEY PORRIDGE.

Take 3 tablespoonfuls of Allinson's barley, mix smoothly with ½ pint of cold water, add ½ pint of boiling milk, and boil 5 to 10 minutes. Pour on shallow plates to cool, then eat with Allinson wholemeal bread, biscuits, rusks, or toast, or stewed fruits.

BARLEY PUDDINGS.

Take 2 tablespoonfuls of Allinson's barley, mix smoothly with a little milk, pour upon it the remainder of 1 pint of milk, flavour and sweeten to taste, boil 2 or 3 minutes, then add 2 eggs lightly beaten, pour into a pie-dish, and bake to a golden brown. Eat with stewed, fresh, or dried fruits.

BARLEY WATER.

Mix smoothly 2 tablespoonfuls of Allinson's barley with a little cold water, then add it to 1 quart of water in a saucepan, and bring to the boil. Pour into a jug, and when cool add the juice of 1 or 2 oranges or lemons. A little sugar may be added when permissible.

BLACK CURRANT TEA.

1 large tablespoonful of black currant jam, 1 pint boiling water. Stir well together, strain when cold, and serve with a little crushed ice if allowed.

BRAN TEA.

Mix 1 oz. of bran with 1 pint of water, boil for ½ hour, strain, and drink cool. A little orange or lemon juice is a pleasant addition. When this is used as a drink at breakfast or tea, a little sugar may be added to it.

BRUNAK.

Take 1-1/2 or 2 teaspoonfuls of Brunak for each large cupful required, mix it with sufficient water, and boil for 2 or 3 minutes to get the full flavour, then strain and add hot milk and sugar to taste. Can be made in a coffee-pot, teapot, or jug if preferred. May be stood on the hob to draw; or if you have any left over from a previous meal it can be boiled up again and served as freshly made.

COCOA.

Put 1 teaspoonful of N.F. cocoa into a breakfast cup; make into a paste with a little cold milk. Fill the cup with milk and water in equal parts, pour into lined saucepan, and boil for 1 minute, stirring carefully. This is best without sugar, and should be given cool.

LEMON WATER.

Squeeze the juice of ½ a Lemon into a tumbler of warm or cold water; add just sufficient sugar to take off the tartness. Or the lemon may be peeled first, then cut in slices, and boiling water poured over them; a little of the peel grated in, and sugar added to taste.

OATMEAL PORRIDGE.

Most people, I think, may know how to make porridge; but it is useful to know that if you take 1 pint of water to each heaped-up breakfastcupful of Allinson breakfast oats, you have just the amount of water for a fairly firm porridge. When the water has boiled, and you have stirred in the oats, place the saucepan on the side of the stove on an asbestos mat. Only an occasional stirring will be required, and there is no fear of burning the porridge. If the porridge is preferred thinner, 1 even cupful to 1 pint of water will be found the proportion.

OATMEAL WATER.

This is very useful in cases of illness, and is a most pleasant drink in hot weather, when it can be flavoured with lemon juice and sweetened a little. To 1 quart of water take 3 oz. of coarse oatmeal or Allinson breakfast oats. Let it simmer gently on the stove for about 2 hours. Then rub it through a fine sieve or gravy strainer; rub it well through, adding a little more hot water when rubbed dry, so as to get all the goodness out of the oatmeal. If it is thick when it has been rubbed through sufficiently, thin it down with water or hot milk—half oatmeal water and half milk is a good mixture. Nothing better can be given to adults or children in cases of colds or feverish attacks. It is nourishing and soothing, and in cases of diarrhoea remedial.

RICE PUDDING.

Wash the rice, put it into a pie-dish, cover with cold water, and bake until the rice is nearly soft throughout. Beat up 1 egg with milk, mix with this a little cinnamon or other flavouring, and pour it over the rice; add sugar to taste, and bake until set.

Sago, tapioca, semolina, and hominy puddings are made after the manner of rice pudding.

DR. ALLINSON'S NATURAL FOOD

FOR BABIES.

(To Prepare the Food.)

Put 1 teaspoonful of the food into a breakfast cup; mix this perfectly smooth with 2 parts milk to 1 of water until the cup is full. Pour into a saucepan and bring to the boil, stirring all the time to prevent it getting lumpy. It is best without sugar, and should be given cool.

FOR INVALIDS AND ADULTS.

Use 3 teaspoonfuls of the food to ½ a pint of milk and water, and prepare as above.

BLANCMANGE.

Mix 6 large tablespoonfuls of the food to a thin paste with a little cold milk, then add 1 quart of milk, flavour with vanilla, lemon or almonds, sweeten to taste; boil 2 or 3 minutes, and pour into wetted mould. Eat with stewed, fresh, or dried fruits, and you have a most nutritious and satisfying dish.

GRUEL.

Mix 1 large tablespoonful of the food with a little cold water, add to this 1 pint of boiling milk and water, boil together a few minutes, take from the fire, let cool, and then eat. A little nutmeg gives a pleasant flavour.

IMPROVED MILK PUDDINGS.

Mix 1 tablespoonful of the food with 1 of rice, sago, tapioca, or hominy, and make as above.

N.B.—The food nicely thickens soups, gravies, &c.

PORRIDGE.

Take 3 tablespoonfuls of the food, mix smoothly, with ½ pint of cold water, add ½ pint boiling milk, and boil 5 or 10 minutes.

Pour on shallow plates to cool, then eat with Allinson wholemeal bread, biscuits, rusks, toast, or stewed fruits.

PUDDINGS.

Take 2 tablespoonfuls of the food, mix smoothly with a little milk, pour upon it the remainder of 1 pint of milk, flavour and sweeten to taste; boil 2 or 3 minutes, then add 2 eggs lightly beaten, pour into a pie-dish, and bake to a golden brown. Eat with stewed, fresh, or dried fruits.

WHOLESOME COOKERY

I.

BREAKFASTS.

As breakfast is the first meal of the day, it must vary in quantity and quality according to the work afterwards to be done. The literary man will best be suited with a light meal, whilst those engaged in hard work will require a heavier one. The clerk, student, business man, or professional man, will find one of the three following breakfasts to suit him well:—

No. I.—Allinson wholemeal bread, 6 to 8 oz., cut thick, with a scrape of butter; with this take from 6 to 8 oz. of ripe, raw fruit, or seasonable green stuff; at the end of the meal have a cup of cool, thin, and not too sweet cocoa, or Brunak, or a cup of cool milk and water, bran tea, or even a cup of water that has been boiled and allowed to go nearly cold. An egg may be taken at this meal by those luxuriously inclined, and if not of a costive habit. The fruits allowed are all the seasonable ones, or dried prunes if there is a tendency to constipation. The green stuffs include watercress, tomatoes, celery, cucumber, and salads. Lettuce must be eaten sparingly at this meal, as it causes a sleepy feeling. Sugar must be used in strict moderation; jam, or fruits stewed with much sugar must be avoided, as they cause mental confusion and disinclination for brain work.

No. II.—3 to 4 oz. of Allinson wholemeal or crushed wheat, coarse oatmeal or groats, hominy, maize or barley meal may be boiled for ½ an hour with milk and water, a very little salt being taken by those who use it. When ready, the porridge should be poured upon platters or soup-plates, allowed to cool, and then eaten with bread. Stewed fruits may be eaten with the porridge, or fresh fruit may be taken afterwards. When porridge is made with water, and then eaten with milk, too much fluid enters the stomach, digestion is delayed, and waterbrash frequently occurs. Meals absorb at least thrice their weight of water in cooking, so that 4 oz. of meal will make at least 16 oz. of porridge. Sugar, syrup, treacle, or molasses should not be eaten with porridge, as they are apt to cause acid risings in the mouth, heartburn, and flatulence. In summer, wholemeal and barleymeal make the best porridges, and they may be taken cold; in autumn, winter, and early spring, oatmeal or hominy are the best, and may be eaten lukewarm. When porridges are eaten, no other course should be taken afterwards, but the entire meal should be made of porridge, bread, and fruit. Neither cocoa nor any other fluids should be taken after a porridge meal, or the stomach becomes filled with too much liquid, and indigestion results. To make the best flavoured porridge, the coarse meal or crushed grain should be stewed in the oven for an hour or two; it may be made the day before it is required, and just warmed through before being brought to the table. This may be eaten with Allinson wholemeal bread and a small quantity of milk, or fresh or stewed fruit.

No. III.—Cut 4 to 6 oz. of Allinson wholemeal bread into dice, put into a basin, and pour over about ½ a pint of boiling milk, or milk and water; cover the basin with a plate, let it stand ten minutes, and then eat slowly. Sugar or salt should not be added to the bread and milk. An apple, pear, orange, grapes, banana, or other seasonable fruit may be eaten afterwards. No other foods should be eaten at this meal, but only the bread, milk, and fruit.

Labourers, artisans, and those engaged in hard physical work may take any of the above breakfasts. If they take No. I., they may allow themselves from 8 to 10 oz. of bread, and should drink a large cup of Brunak afterwards, as their work requires a fair amount of liquid to carry off some of the heat caused by the burning up of food whilst they are at work. If No. II. breakfast is taken, 6 to 8 oz. of meal may be allowed. If No. III. breakfast is eaten, then 6 or 8 oz. of bread and 2 pint of milk may be taken.

N.B.—Women require about a quarter less food than men do, and must arrange the quantity accordingly.

II.

MIDDAY MEALS.

The meal in the middle of the day must vary according to the work to be done after it. If much mental strain has to be borne or business done, the meal must be a light one, and should be lunch rather than dinner. Those engaged in hard physical work should make their chief meal about midday, and have a light repast in the evening.

LUNCH.—One of the simplest lunches is that composed of Allinson wholemeal bread and fruit. From 6 to 8 oz. of bread may be eaten, and about ½ lb. of any raw fruit that is in season; afterwards a glass of lemon water or bran tea, Brunak, or a cup of thin, cool, and not too sweet cocoa may be taken, or a tumbler of milk and water slowly sipped. The fruit may be advantageously replaced by a salad, which is a pleasant change from fruit, and sits as lightly on the stomach. Wholemeal biscuits and fruit, with a cup of fluid, form another good lunch. A basin of any kind of porridge with milk, but without sugar, also makes a light and good midday repast; or a basin of thin vegetable soup and bread, or macaroni, or even plain vegetables. The best lunch of all will be found in Allinson wholemeal bread, and salad or fruit, as it is not wise to burden the system with too much cooked food, and one never feels so light after made dishes as after bread and fruit.

Labouring men who wish to take something with them to work will find 12 oz. of Allinson wholemeal bread, ½ lb. fresh fruit, and a large mug of Brunak or cocoa satisfy them well; or instead of cocoa they may have milk and water, lemon water, lemonade, oatmeal water, or some harmless non-alcoholic drink. Another good meal is made from ½ lb. of the wholemeal bread and butter, and a ¼ lb. of peas pudding spread between the slices. The peas can be flavoured with a little pepper, salt, and mustard by those who still cling to condiments. 12 oz. of the wholemeal bread, 2 or 3 oz. of cheese, some raw fruit, or an onion, celery, watercress, or other greenstuff, with a large cup of fluid, form another good meal. ½ lb. of coarse oatmeal or crushed wheat made into porridge the day before, and warmed up at midday, will last a man well until he gets home at night. Or a boiled bread pudding may be taken to work, warmed and eaten. This is made from the wholemeal bread, which is soaked in hot water until soft, then crushed or crumbled, some currants or raisins are then mixed with this, a little soaked sago stirred in; lastly, a very little sugar and spice are added as a flavouring. This mixture is then tied up in a pudding cloth and boiled, or it may be put in a pudding basin covered with a cloth, and boiled in a saucepan. A pleasing addition to this pudding is some finely chopped almonds, or Brazil nuts.

III.

DINNERS.

As dinner is the chief meal of the day it should consist of substantial food. It may be taken in the middle of the day by those who work hard; but if taken at night, at least five hours must elapse before going to bed, so that the stomach may have done its work before sleep comes on.

A dinner may consist of many courses or different dishes, but the simpler the dishes and the less numerous the courses the better. A person who makes his meal from one dish only is the wisest of all. He who limits himself to two courses does well, but he who takes more than three courses lays up for himself stomach troubles or disorder of the system. When only one course is had, then good solid food must be eaten; when two courses are the rule, a moderate amount of each should be taken; and it three different dishes are provided, a proportionately lighter quantity of each. Various dishes may be served for the dinner meal, such as soups, omelettes, savouries, pies, batters, and sweet courses.

The plainest dinner any one can eat is that composed of Allinson wholemeal bread and raw fruit. A man in full work may eat from 12 to 16 oz. of the wholemeal bread, and about the same quantity of ripe raw fruit. The bread is best dry, the next best is when a thin scrape of butter is spread on it. If hard physical work has to be done, a cup of Brunak, cocoa, milk and water, or lemon water, should be drunk at the end of the meal. In winter these fluids might be taken warmed, but in summer they are best cool or cold. This wholesome fare can be varied in a variety of ways; some might like a salad instead of the fruit, and others may prefer cold vegetables. A few Brazil nuts, almonds, walnuts, some Spanish nuts, or a piece of cocoanut may be eaten with the bread in winter. Others not subject to piles, constipation, or eczema, &c., may take 2 oz. of cheese and an onion with their bread, or a hard-boiled egg. This simple meal can be easily carried to work, or on a journey. Wholemeal biscuits or Allinson rusks may be used instead of bread if one is on a walking tour, cycling trip, or boating excursion, or even on ordinary occasions for a change.

Of cooked dinners, the simplest is that composed of potatoes baked, steamed, or boiled in their skins, eaten with another vegetable, sauce, and the wholemeal bread. Baked potatoes are the most wholesome, and their skins should always be eaten; steamed potatoes are next; whilst boiled ones, especially if peeled, are not nearly so good. Any seasonable vegetable may be steamed and eaten with the potatoes, such as cauliflower, cabbage, sprouts, broccoli, carrot, turnip, beetroot, parsnips, or boiled celery, or onions. Recipes for the sauces used with this course will be found in another part of the book; they may be parsley, onion, caper, tomato, or brown gravy sauce. This dinner may be varied by adding to it a poached, fried, or boiled egg. As a second course, baked apples, or stewed fresh fruit and bread may be eaten; or Allinson bread pudding, or rice, sago, tapioca, or macaroni pudding with stewed fruit. Persons troubled with piles, varicose veins, varicocele, or constipation must avoid this dinner as much as possible. If they do eat it they must be sure to eat the skins of the potatoes, and take the Allinson bread pudding or bread and fruit afterwards, avoiding puddings of rice, sago, tapioca, or macaroni.

IV.

EVENING MEAL.

Evening meal or tea meal should be the last meal at which solid food is eaten. It should always be a light one, and the later it is eaten the less substantial it should be. Heavy or hard work after tea is no excuse for a supper. This meal must be taken at least three hours before retiring. From 4 to 6 oz. of Allinson wholemeal bread may be allowed with a poached or lightly boiled egg, a salad, or fruit, or some kind of green food. The fluid drunk may be Brunak, cocoa, milk and water, bran tea, or even plain water, boiled and taken cool. Those who are restless at night, nervous, or sleepless must not drink tea at this meal. Fruit in the evening is not considered good, and when taken it should be cooked rather than raw. Boiled celery will be found to be lighter on the stomach at this meal than the raw vegetable. When it is boiled, as little water as possible should be used; the water that the celery is boiled in may be thickened with Allinson fine wheatmeal, made into sauce, and poured over the cooked celery; by this means we do not loose the valuable salts dissolved out of the food by boiling. Mustard and cress, watercress, radishes, and spring onions may be eaten if the evening meal is taken 4 or 5 hours before going to bed. Those who are away from home all day, and who take their food to their work may have some kind of milk pudding at this meal. Wheatmeal blancmange, or cold milk pudding may occasionally be eaten those who are costive will find a boiled onion or some braized onions very useful. Boil the onion in as little water as possible and serve up with the liquor it is boiled in. To prepare braized onions, fry them first until nicely brown, using butter or olive oil, then add a cupful of boiling water to the contents of the frying pan, cover with a plate, and let cook for an hour. This is not really a rich food, but one easy of digestion and of great use to the sleepless. Those who want to rise early must make their last meal a light one. Those troubled with dreams or restlessness must do the same. Very little fluid should be taken last thing at night, as it causes persons to rise frequently to empty the bladder.

V.

SUPPERS.

Hygienic livers will never take such meals, even if tea has been early, or hard work done since the tea meal was taken. No solid food must be eaten. The most that should be consumed is a cup of Brunak, cocoa, lemon water, bran tea, or even boiled water, but never milk. In winter warm drinks may be taken, and in summer cool ones.

VI.

DRINKS.

LEMON WATER is made by squeezing the juice of ½ a lemon into a tumbler of warm or cold water; to this is added just enough sugar to take off the tartness. Some peel the lemon first, then cut in slices, pour boiling water over the slices, grate in a little of the peel, and add sugar to taste.

BRUNAK.—Take 1-1/2 to 2 teaspoonfuls of Brunak for each large cupful required, mix it with sufficient water, and boil for 2 or 3 minutes to get the full flavour, then strain and add hot milk and sugar to taste. Can be made in a coffee-pot, teapot, or jug if preferred. May be stood on the hob to draw; or it you have any left over from a previous meal it can be boiled up again and served as freshly made.

COCOA.—This is best made by putting a teaspoonful of any good cocoa, such as Allinson's, into a breakfast cup; boiling water is then poured upon this and stirred; 1 tablespoonful of milk must be added to each cup, and 1 teaspoonful of sugar where sugar is used, or 1 or 2 teaspoonfuls of condensed milk and no extra sugar.

BRAN TEA.—Mix 1 oz. of bran with 1 pint of water; boil for ½ an hour, strain, and drink cool. A little orange or lemon juice is a pleasant addition. When this is used as a drink at breakfast or tea, a little milk and sugar may be added to it.

CHOCOLATE.—Allow 1 bar of Allinson's chocolate for each cup of fluid. Break the chocolate in bits, put into a saucepan, add a little boiling water, put on the fire, and stir until the chocolate is dissolved, then add rest of fluid and boil 2 or 3 minutes. Pour the chocolate into cups, and add about 1 tablespoonful of fresh milk to each cup, but no extra sugar. The milk may be added to the chocolate whilst boiling, if desired.

WHOLEMEAL COOKERY

Most of my readers have received great benefit from eating wholemeal bread instead of white, and they may all gain further good it they will use Allinson wholemeal flour in place of white for all cooking purposes. Those who are at all constipated, or who suffer from piles, varicose veins, varicocele, back pain, &c., should never use white flour in cooking. Those who are inclined to stoutness should use wholemeal flour rather than white. Hygienists and health-reformers should not permit white flour to enter their houses, unless it is to make bill-stickers' paste or some like stuff. Toothless children must not be given any food but milk and water until they cut at least two teeth.

Every kind of cookery can be done with wholemeal flour. In making ordinary white sauce or vegetable sauce, this is how we make it; Chop fine some onion or parsley; boil in a small quantity of water, stir in wholemeal flour and milk, add a little pepper and salt, thin with hot water, and thus produce a sauce that helps down vegetables and potatoes. In making a brown sauce we put a little butter or olive oil in the frying-pan; let it bubble and sputter, dredge in Allinson wholemeal flour, stir it round with a knife until browned, add boiling water, pepper, salt, a little ketchup, and you then have a nice brown sauce for many dishes. If we wish to make it very tasty we fry a finely chopped onion first and add that to it. White sweet sauce is made from wholemeal flour, milk, sugar, and a little cinnamon, cloves, lemon juice, vanilla, or other flavouring. Yorkshire puddings, Norfolk dumplings, batter puddings, and such puddings can all be made with wholemeal flour, and are more nourishing and healthy, and do not lie so heavy as those made from white flour. Pancakes can be made from wholemeal flour just as well as from white.

All kinds of pastry, pie-crusts, under crusts, &c., are best made from Allinson wholemeal, and if much butter, lard, or dripping is used they will lie just as heavy, and cause heartburn just as much as those made with white flour. There is a substitute for pie-crusts that is very tasty, and not at all harmful. We call it "batter," and it can be used for savoury dishes as well as sweet ones.

SAVOURY DISHES MADE WITH BATTER.

Fry some potatoes, then some onions, put them in layers in a pie-dish; next make a batter of Allinson wholemeal flour, 1 or 2 eggs, milk, and a little pepper with salt; pour over the fried vegetables as they lie in the dish, bake in the oven from ½ an hour to 1 hour, until, in fact, the batter has formed a crust; eat with the usual vegetables. Or chop fine cold vegetables of any kind, fry onions and add to them, put in a pie-dish, pour some of the batter as above over them, and bake. All kinds of cold vegetables, cold soup, porridge, &c., can go into this, and tinned or fresh tomatoes will make it more savoury. Tomatoes may be wiped, put in a pie-dish, batter poured over, and then baked, and are very tasty this way. Butter adds to the flavour of these dishes, but does not make them more wholesome or more nourishing.

STEWED FRUIT PUDDING.

Cut Allinson wholemeal bread into slices a little over a ¼ of an inch thick, line a pie-dish with these, having first cut off the hard crusts. Then fill the dish with hot stewed fruit of any kind, and at once cover it with a layer of bread, gently pressed on the hot fruit. Turn out when cold on to a flat dish, pour over it a white sauce, and serve.

SUBSTANTIAL BREAD PUDDINGS.

Soak crusts or slices of Allinson bread in hot water, then break fine in a pie-dish, add to this soaked currants, raisins, chopped nuts or almonds, a beaten-up egg, and milk, with sugar and spice, and bake in the oven. Or tie the whole up in a pudding-cloth and boil. Serve with white sauce or eat with stewed fresh fruit. These puddings can be eaten hot or cold; labourers can take them to their work for dinner, and their children cannot have a better meal to take to school.

SWEET BATTER.

Mix Allinson wholemeal flour, milk, 1 or 2 eggs together, and a little sugar and cinnamon, and it is ready for use. Stew ripe cherries, gooseberries, currants, raspberries, plums, damsons, or other ripe fruit in a jar, pour into a pie-dish; pour into the batter named above, bake, and this is a good substitute for a fruit pie. Prunes can be treated the same way, or the batter can be cooked in the saucepan, poured into a mould, allowed to go cold and set; then it forms wholemeal blancmange, and may be eaten with stewed fresh fruit. Rusks, cheesecakes, buns, biscuits, and other like articles as Madeira cake, pound cake, wedding cake, &c., can all be made of wholemeal flour.

WHOLEMEAL SOUP.

Chop fine any kinds of greens or vegetables, stew in a little water until thoroughly done, then add plenty of hot water, with pepper and salt to taste, and a ¼ of an hour before serving, pour in a cupful of the "Sweet Batter," and you get a thick, nourishing soup. To make it more savoury, fry your vegetables before making into soup.

A MONTH'S MENUS FOR ONE PERSON.

No. 1.

CAULIFLOWER SOUP.

½ small cauliflower, ½ pint milk and water, small piece of butter, 1 teaspoonful of fine wholemeal, pepper and salt to taste. Wash and cut up the cauliflower, cook till tender with the milk and water, add butter and seasoning; smooth the meal with a little water, thicken the soup with it, boil up for a minute and serve.

WHOLEMEAL BATTER.

2 oz. wholemeal, 1 gill of milk, 1 egg, seasoning to taste. Make a batter of the ingredients, butter a flat tin or a small pie-dish, turn the batter into it, and bake it from 20 to 30 minutes. Eat with vegetables.

BLANCMANGE.

1 even dessertspoonful of wheatmeal, 1 ditto cornflour, ¼ pint milk, sugar and vanilla to taste. Smooth the meal and cornflour with a little of the milk, bring the rest to the boil, stir in the mixture, add flavouring, let it all simmer

for 5 to 8 minutes, stirring all the time. Pour into a wetted mould, and turn out when cold.

No. 2.

ARTICHOKE SOUP.

¼ lb. artichokes, ¼ lb. potatoes, ¾ pint milk and water (equal parts), ¼ oz. butter, pepper and salt to taste. Peel, wash, and cut up small the vegetables, and cook them in the milk and water, until tender. Rub them through a sieve, return to saucepan, add butter and seasoning, boil up and serve.

FLAGOLETS.

3 oz. of flagolets, ¼ pint parsley sauce. Cook the flagolets till tender, season with pepper and salt, and serve with the sauce. Make it as follows; 1 gill of milk, 1 teaspoonful of cornflour, 1 teaspoonful of finely chopped parsley, pepper and salt, and a small bit of butter. Boil up the milk, thicken with the cornflour, previously smoothed with a spoonful of water; boil up, season, and mix with the parsley before serving.

WHEATMEAL PUDDING.

2 oz. of fine wheatmeal, 1 egg, ½ gill of milk, 1 tablespoonful sultanas washed and picked, ½ oz. of oiled butter, a little grated lemon peel, sugar to taste. Beat up the egg and mix well all ingredients; butter a small pie-dish, and bake the pudding about ½ hour.

No. 3.

CARROT SOUP.

1 carrot, 1 potato, and 1 small onion cut up small, 1 pint of water, a little butter, and pepper and salt to taste. Cook the vegetables in the water till quite tender, rub them through a sieve, adding a little water if necessary; return to saucepan, add seasoning and butter, boil up and serve.

LENTIL CAKES.

2 oz. of picked and washed Egyptian lentils, 1 small finely chopped and fried onion, 1 dessertspoonful of cold boiled vermicelli, 1 egg, some breadcrumbs, seasoning to taste. Stew the lentils with the onion in just enough water to cover them; when cooked, they should be a thick purée. Season to taste, add the vermicelli, and form into 1 or 2 cakes, dip in egg and breadcrumb, and fry in vege-butter, or butter. Serve with potatoes and green vegetables.

TAPIOCA PUDDING.

1 oz. small tapioca, ½ pint of milk, sugar to taste. Put the tapioca into a small pie-dish, let it soak in a very little water for half an hour, pour off any which has not been absorbed. Pour the milk over the soaked tapioca, and bake it in the oven until thoroughly cooked. Eat with or without stewed fruit.

No. 4.

CLEAR SOUP (Julienne).

¾ pint vegetable stock, 1 tablespoonful dried Julienne (vegetables), a little butter, pepper and salt to taste. Cook the Julienne in the stock until tender, add butter and seasoning and serve.

HAGGIS.

2 oz. of wheatmeal, 1 oz. of rolled oatmeal, 1 egg, ¼ oz. of oiled butter, ½ gill milk, a teaspoonful of grated onion, a pinch of herbs, pepper and salt to taste. Beat up the egg, mix it with the milk, and add the other ingredients. Turn the mixture into a small greased basin, and steam the haggis 1-1/2 hours. Serve with vegetables.

GROUND RICE PUDDING.

1 oz. of ground rice, a scanty ½ pint of milk, sugar and flavouring to taste, ½ egg. Boil the milk, stir the ground rice into it; let it simmer for 10 minutes, then add sugar and flavouring and the ½ egg well beaten; turn the mixture into a small pie-dish, and bake in the oven until a golden colour.

No. 5.

CLEAR TOMATO SOUP.

2 tablespoonfuls of tinned tomatoes, or 1 fair-sized fresh one, 1 small finely chopped and fried onion, a teaspoonful of vermicelli, pepper and salt to taste, ½ pint of water. Boil the tomatoes with the onion and water for 5 to 10 minutes, then drain all the liquid; return to the saucepan, season and sprinkle in the vermicelli, let the soup cook until the vermicelli is soft, and serve.

MACARONI WITH CHEESE.

2 oz. of macaroni or Spaghetti, a little grated cheese, pepper and salt to taste. Boil the

macaroni in as much water as it will absorb (about ½ pint). Season to taste. When tender serve with grated cheese and vegetables.

WHEATMEAL BATTER.

2 oz. of meal, 1 oz. of desiccated cocoanut, 1 gill of milk, 1 egg, sugar to taste, ¼ oz. of oiled butter. Make a batter of the egg, milk, and meal, add the other ingredients, and bake the batter in a small buttered pie-dish.

No. 6.

LENTIL SOUP.

2 oz. of Egyptian lentils, 2 oz. each of carrots and turnips cut up small, ½ oz. of onion chopped fine, ½ oz. of butter, seasoning to taste, 1 pint of water. Cook the vegetables and lentils in the water until quite tender, then rub them through a sieve. Return to the saucepan, add butter and seasoning, boil up, and serve with sippets of toast.

RICE AND TOMATOES.

¼ lb. rice, ½ pint water, ¼ oz. of butter, pepper and salt to taste, 1 large tomato or two small ones. Set the rice over the fire with the water (cold) and the butter and seasoning; let it simmer until the water is absorbed and the rice fairly tender. It will take 20 minutes. Meanwhile place the tomatoes in a small dish, sprinkle with pepper and salt, place a little bit of butter on each, a few spoonfuls of water in the dish, and bake them from 15 to 25 minutes. Spread the rice on a flat dish, place the tomatoes in the middle, pour the juice over, and serve.

WHEATMEAL AND SAGO PUDDING.

1 dessertspoonful of sago, 1 ditto of wheatmeal, ½ pint milk, sugar and flavouring to taste. Boil the sago and wheatmeal in the milk until the sago is well swelled out. Flavour to taste, pour the mixture into a little pie-dish, and bake the pudding until a golden colour.

No. 7.

POTATO SOUP.

½ lb. of potatoes, 1 pint of water, 1 small onion, a piece of celery, a little piece of butter, a teaspoonful of chopped parsley, pepper and salt to taste. Peel, wash, and cut up small the vegetables, and cook them in the water till quite tender. Rub the mixture through a sieve, add the butter and seasoning, boil up, mix in the parsley, and serve.

CAULIFLOWER AU GRATIN.

1 small cauliflower, 1 oz. of grated cheese, 1 tablespoonful of breadcrumbs, ½ oz. of butter, pepper and salt. Boil the cauliflower until tender, cut it up and arrange it in a small pie-dish; sprinkle over the cheese and breadcrumbs, dust with pepper and salt, place the butter in little bits over the top, and bake the cauliflower until golden brown. Serve with white sauce. (See "Sauces.")

APPLE PIE.

2 medium-sized cooking apples, sugar and cinnamon or lemon peel to taste. Some paste for short crust. Pare, core, and cut up the apples, and fill a small pie-dish with them; add sugar and cinnamon to taste, and a little water. Cover with paste, and bake in a fairly

quick oven until brown, then let cook gently for another ¼ hour in a cooler part of the oven.

No. 8.

POTATO SOUP (2).

2 medium-sized potatoes, 1 small onion chopped fine, and fried a nice brown in butter or vege-butter, ¼ pint milk, ¾ pint water, 1 piece of celery, pepper and salt to taste. Peel, wash, and cut up the potatoes, and cut up the celery. Boil with the water until tender. Rub the vegetables through a sieve, return the soup to the saucepan, add seasoning, milk, and onion; boil up and serve.

SWEET CORN TART.

2 tablespoonfuls of tinned sweet corn, ¼ oz. of butter, pepper and salt to taste, 1 egg, some paste for crust. Beat up the egg and mix with the sweet corn, season to taste. Roll out the paste and line a plate with it, turn the sweet corn mixture on to the paste, and bake the tart until a light brown. Serve with brown sauce or tomato sauce.

RICE PUDDING.

1 oz. of rice, ½ pint of milk, sugar and flavouring to taste. Wash the rice and put it into a pie-dish. Bring the milk to the boil, pour it over the rice, add the sugar and any kind of flavouring, and bake the pudding till the rice is tender.

No. 9.

RICE CHEESE SOUP.

1 dessertspoonful of rice, ¾ pint water, ¼ pint milk, 1 oz. grated cheese, ¼ oz. butter, seasoning to taste. Cook the rice in the milk and water until tender, then add the cheese, butter, and seasoning, and let the soup boil up until the cheese is dissolved.

VEGETABLE PIE.

2 oz. each of potato, carrot, turnip, celery, tomato (or any other vegetable in season), a small onion, ½ oz. of butter, pepper and salt to taste, 1 teaspoonful of sago. Chop fine the onion and fry it. Boil all the vegetables, previously washed and cut up, in ½ pint of water. When they are quite tender, put all in a pie-dish, adding seasoning to taste. Add enough water for gravy, and sprinkle in the sago. Cover with short crust, and bake in a moderately hot oven.

STEWED PRUNES AND GRATED COCOANUT.

Stew some Californian plums in enough water to cover them well. If possible, they should be soaked over night. Grate some fresh cocoanut, after removing the brown outer skin, and serve separately.

No. 10.

ASPARAGUS SOUP.

½ dozen sticks of asparagus, ½ pint water, ¼ pint milk, 1 level dessertspoonful of cornflour, ¼ oz. of butter, pepper and salt to taste. Boil the asparagus in the water till tender, add the seasoning, and the cornflour smoothed in the milk, boil up and serve.

MACARONI WITH CAPER SAUCE.

2 oz. macaroni, ¼ pint white sauce (see "Sauces"); 1 teaspoonful capers chopped small, enough of the caper vinegar to taste. Boil the macaroni in ½ pint of water until tender. Make the white sauce, then add the capers and vinegar. Serve with vegetables.

PRUNE BATTER.

8 or 10 well-cooked Californian plums, with a little of the juice, 2 oz. of fine wheatmeal, ½ oz. of butter, 1 gill of milk, and 1 egg. Make a batter of the milk, meal, and egg, oil the butter, and stir it in. Place the prunes in a little pie-dish, pour the batter over, and bake until a nice brown.

No. 11.

TOMATO SOUP.

1 teacupful of tinned tomatoes, or 6 oz. of fresh ones, 1 teaspoonful of cornflour, 1 small onion, pepper and salt to taste, and a little butter. Chop the onion up fine, and cook the tomatoes and onion in enough water to make ½ pint of soup. When cooked 15 minutes rub the vegetables through a sieve; return to the saucepan, boil up, thicken with the cornflour smoothed with a spoonful of water, and add a little piece of butter; serve with sippets of toast.

BREAD STEAK.

One slice of Wholemeal bread, a small finely chopped onion, a little milk, half an egg beaten up, pepper and salt, a little piece of butter. Dip the bread in milk, then in egg; melt the butter in a frying pan, fry the bread and onion a nice brown, sprinkle with seasoning and serve with potato and greens.

SEMOLINA PUDDING.

1 oz. of semolina, ½ pint of milk, sugar and vanilla to taste. Boil the semolina in the milk until well thickened, add sugar and flavouring, pour the mixture into a little pie-dish, and bake until a golden colour.

No. 12.

BREAD SOUP.

1 slice of Allinson bread, 1 small finely chopped onion fried brown, a pinch of nutmeg, pepper and salt to taste. Boil the bread in ¾ pint of water and milk in equal parts, adding the onion and seasoning. When the bread is quite tender, rub all through a sieve, return soup to the saucepan, boil up, and serve.

RICE AND MUSHROOMS.

¼ lb. of rice, ¼ lb. of mushrooms, a little butter and seasoning. Cook the rice in ½ pint of water, as directed in recipe for "Rice." Peel and wash the mushrooms, place them in a flat tin with a few spoonfuls of water, a dusting of pepper and salt and a bit of butter on each. Bake them from 15 to 20 minutes, spread the rice on a flat dish, place the mushrooms in the middle, pour over the gravy, and serve.

BREAD PUDDING.

3 oz. of bread, 1 oz. sultanas, ½ doz. sweet almonds chopped fine, 1 well-beaten egg,

cinnamon and sugar to taste, ½ oz. of butter, a little milk. Soak the bread in milk, and squeeze the surplus out with a spoon. Mix all the ingredients together, add the butter oiled, pour the mixture into a buttered pie-dish, and bake the pudding from 30 to 45 minutes.

No. 13.

ONION SOUP.

1 small Spanish onion, 1 medium-sized potato, ¼ oz. of butter, pepper and salt and a pinch of mixed herbs, a little milk. Cut up the vegetables and cook them in ½ pint of water, adding a little herbs. When tender, rub the vegetables through a sieve, return the soup to the saucepan, add the butter and seasoning, and serve.

MACARONI AND TOMATOES.

2 oz, of macaroni, ½ teacupful tinned tomatoes, 1-1/2 gills of water, a little grated cheese. Cook the rice in the water and tomatoes until tender, add seasoning, and serve with grated cheese and vegetables.

STEAMED PUDDING.

2 oz. wheatmeal, 1 oz. of sago, 1 egg, ½ oz. of oiled butter, 1 oz. sultanas, ½ saltspoonful of cinnamon, sugar to taste. Soak the sago over the fire in a little water; when almost tender drain off any water that is not absorbed, mix it with the other ingredients, pour the mixture into a soup-or small basin, tie with a cloth, and steam the pudding for an hour. Serve with white sauce.

GREEN PEA SOUP.

½ teacupful green peas, ¼ oz. of butter, 1 spray of mint, a teaspoonful of fine meal, a little milk, pepper and salt to taste. Boil the green peas in ½ pint of water, adding seasoning and the mint. When the peas are tender, take out the mint, add the butter, smooth the meal with a little milk, and thicken the soup. Let it cook for 2 to 3 minutes, and serve.

VERMICELLI RISSOLES.

2 ozs. of vermicelli, 1 oz. of grated cheese, 1 egg well beaten, a few breadcrumbs, seasoning to taste, 1 gill of water, a little butter, or vege-butter. Boil the vermicelli in the water until tender and all the water absorbed. Then add seasoning, the egg, the cheese, and a few breadcrumbs, if the mixture is too moist. Form into 2 or 3 little cakes, place little bits of butter on each, and bake them a golden brown.

TRIFLE.

2 sponge cakes, 1 gill of custard, a little jam, a few ratafias, ½ oz. of chopped almond. Cut the sponge cakes in half, spread them with jam, arranging them in a little pie-dish, sprinkling crumbled ratafias and the almonds between the pieces of cake. Pour the custard over, let it all soak for half an hour, and serve.

SPLIT PEA SOUP.

2 oz. of split peas cooked overnight, 3 oz. of potatoes cut into pieces, a piece of celery, a slice of Spanish onion chopped up, seasoning to taste. Soak the peas in water overnight, after picking them over and washing them. Set them over the fire in the morning, and cook them with the vegetables till quite tender. Then rub all through a sieve. Return to the saucepan, add pepper and salt, and a little water if necessary; boil up, and serve with sippets of toast.

HOT-POT.

½ lb. potatoes, 3 oz. Spanish onion peeled and sliced, ½ teacupful tomatoes, ½ oz. of butter, pepper and salt to taste. Arrange the potatoes, onions, and tomatoes in layers in a small pie-dish, and sprinkle pepper and salt between the vegetables. Cut the butter in little bits, and scatter them over the top. Fill the dish with boiling water, and boil the hot-pot for 1 to 1-1/2 hours, adding a little hot water if needed.

BAKED APPLES AND WHITE SAUCE.

Wash and core a good-sized apple, fill the core with 1 or 2 stoned dates, and bake it in the oven in a dish or tin with a few spoonfuls of water until well done. Serve with sauce.

No. 16.

LEEK SOUP.

1 leek, ¼ lb. potatoes, ½ pint water, 1 gill of milk, ¼ oz. of butter, pepper and salt to taste. Peel, wash, and cut up the leek and potatoes, and cook them till tender in the water. Then rub the vegetables through a sieve. Return to

the saucepan, add the milk, butter, and seasoning, boil up, and serve.

SAVOURY CUSTARD.

1-1/2 gills of milk, 1 egg, 1 oz. of grated cheese, a pinch of nutmeg, pepper and salt to taste. Proceed as in savoury custard, and serve with potatoes and greens.

CHOCOLATE BLANCMANGE.

½ pint of milk, 1 teaspoonful N.F. cocoa, 1 oz. of half cornflour and fine wheatmeal, sugar and vanilla essence to taste. Bring the milk to the boil, mix cocoa, flour, and wheatmeal, and smooth them with a little water. Stir the mixture into the boiling milk, sweeten and flavour, keep stirring, and allow to cook 5 minutes. Pour into a wetted mould, and allow to get cold. Turn out, and serve.

No. 17.

TURNIP SOUP.

¼ lb. turnip, a small onion, and 2 oz. of potato, a little butter and seasoning, ½ pint water. Wash, peel, and cut up the vegetables, and cook them in the water until tender. Rub them through a sieve, return the mixture to the saucepan, add butter and seasoning, boil up, and serve.

POTATO BATTER.

1 gill of milk, 1 egg, 2 oz. wheatmeal, 1 oz. of vege-butter, 6 oz. cold boiled potatoes. Fry the potatoes in the butter, make a batter of the milk, meal, and egg, mix it with the potatoes, add seasoning, pour the mixture in a little pie-dish, and bake the savoury for half an hour.

LEMON MOULD.

1 oz. of tapioca, ½ pint of water, juice and rind of ¼ lemon, 1 large tablespoonful of golden syrup. Boil the tapioca until quite tender, with the Lemon rind, in the water. Take out the rind, add the syrup and lemon juice, mix well, pour the mixture into a wetted mould, turn out when cold, and serve.

No. 18.

APPLE SOUP.

1 large cooking apple, 1 small finely chopped onion, seasoning and sugar to taste, a little butter, 1 teaspoonful of cornflour, ½ pint of water. Peel and cut up the apple, and cook with the onion in the water till quite tender. Rub the mixture through a sieve, return to the saucepan, add the butter, seasoning and sugar, thicken the soup with the cornflour, and serve.

RICE CHEESECAKES.

2 oz. rice, 1 gill water, 1 oz. of grated cheese, seasoning, a pinch of nutmeg, 1 egg, a little wheatmeal, and some vege-butter, or butter. Cook the rice in the water until quite dry and soft, mix the egg—well beaten—seasoning, and cheese with the rice, and form the mixture into small cakes. Roll in wheatmeal, and fry them a golden brown. Serve with vegetables and brown sauce.

PLUM PIE.

½ lb. ripe plums, sugar to taste, some paste. Wash the plums and put them in a small pie-dish, pour ½ teacupful of water over them, add sugar, cover the plums with a short crust, and bake the pie a golden brown.

No. 19.

CELERY SOUP.

½ stick celery, ½ small onion, ¼ oz. butter, 1 potato, pepper and salt. Wash, peel, and cut up the vegetables, and cook them in ½ pint of water till tender. Rub through a sieve, return to the saucepan, season with pepper and salt, add the butter, boil up, and serve.

APPLE AND ONION PIE.

6 oz. apples, ¼ lb. Spanish onions, 1 hard-boiled egg, a little butter, pepper and salt to taste, some paste for a short crust. Peel and cut up the apples and onion, stew gently with a little water. When nearly tender, season and add the butter, turn the mixture into a small pie-dish, quarter the egg, and place the pieces on the mixture, cover with a crust, and bake the pie ½ hour.

MACARONI PUDDING.

2 oz. macaroni, ½ pint milk, 6 eggs, sugar and flavouring to taste. Boil the macaroni in water until tender. Cut into little pieces and place in a little pie-dish; beat the milk, add the egg, well beaten, carefully with it, add sugar and flavouring, pour the custard over the macaroni, and bake until set. Serve with stewed fruit.

No. 20.

BUTTER BEAN SOUP.

2 oz. of butter beans soaked overnight in 1 pint of water, ½ small onion cut up small, 2 oz. carrot, 2 oz. celery, ½ oz. butter. Cook all the vegetables until tender, adding water as it boils away. When all is tender, rub the vegetables through a sieve, return to the saucepan, season with pepper and salt, add the butter, boil up the soup, and serve.

SAUSAGES.

1 teacupful of breadcrumbs, 1 egg well beaten, ½ small onion chopped fine, ½ saltspoonful of herbs, ½ oz. butter, seasoning to taste. Oil the butter and mix it with the breadcrumbs, egg, onion, herbs, and seasoning. Make the mixture into sausages, roll them into a little breadcrumb, and fry them brown in a little vege-butter.

ROLLED WHEAT PUDDING.

1 oz. rolled wheat, ½ pint milk, 1 tablespoonful of currants and sultanas mixed, sugar to taste. Cook the rolled wheat in the milk for fifteen minutes, then add the fruit, and let simmer another 15 minutes. Pour the mixture into a small pie-dish, and bake in the oven until golden brown.

No. 21.

FRENCH SOUP.

1 small onion chopped fine, 1 oz. of cheese shredded fine, 1 slice of dry toast, ¾ pint of water, a little milk, pepper and salt to taste. Break up the toast, and set all the ingredients over the fire; cook till the onion is tender, add ½ gill of milk, and serve.

VEGETABLE PIE.

½ lb. potatoes, peeled and cut in pieces, ½ Spanish onion chopped up, 1 tomato, ½ oz. butter, pepper and salt, some paste for crust. Stew the potatoes and onion in a little water; when tender, cut up the tomato and mix it in, season and add the butter; place the vegetables in a small pie-dish, cover with paste, and bake ½ hour or until golden brown.

CHOCOLATE PUDDING.

½ oz. ground rice, ½ pint milk, 1 teaspoonful N.F. cocoa, a little vanilla, sugar to taste, and 1 egg. Boil the rice in the milk for 5 minutes, let it cool a little, mix in the egg, well-beaten, cocoa, sugar, and vanilla. Pour the mixture into a small pie-dish, and bake for 20 to 30 minutes.

No. 22.

SORREL SOUP.

1 potato, 1 small onion, 1 good handful of sorrel washed and chopped fine, a little butter, pepper and salt, ½ pint water, 1 gill milk. Peel, wash, and cut up the potatoes and onion, boil in the water till tender, and rub through a sieve. Return the mixture to the saucepan, add the milk, sorrel, butter, and seasoning. Simmer gently for 10 minutes, and serve.

SAVOURY BATTER.

2 oz. fine wheatmeal, 1 gill of milk, 1 egg, 1 teaspoonful finely chopped parsley, ½ small grated onion, ¼ oz. butter, pepper and salt. Make a batter of the meal, egg, and milk, mix in the other ingredients, pour the mixture into a buttered pie-dish, and bake the batter ½ hour.

STEWED FRUIT AND CUSTARD.

Any kind of stewed fruit. *Custard*: 1 gill of milk, sugar and vanilla to taste, and 1 egg. Heat the milk, beat up the egg, and stir the milk into it gradually; pour the mixture into a small jug, place this in a saucepan of fast-boiling water, keep stirring until the spoon gets coated, which shows that the custard is thickening. Remove the saucepan from the fire immediately, and continue stirring the custard until it is well thickened. Then cool it, placing the jug in cold water. When cold, serve with stewed fruit.

No. 23.

GREEN PEA SOUP.

½ teacupful green peas, 1 or 2 finely chopped spring onions, a little butter, pepper and salt, a dessertspoonful of meal, and 1 gill of milk. Cook the green peas and spring onions in ½ pint of water until quite tender. Add the butter and seasoning, thicken the soup with the meal (which should be smoothed with the milk), and boil the soup for a minute or two before serving.

MUSHROOM TARTLETS.

¼ lb. mushrooms, ½ oz. butter, pepper and salt, ½ oz. vermicelli, cooked and cold, a little paste for short crust. Stew the mushrooms in the butter, after having dried them and cut into pieces. When they are cooked mix them well with the vermicelli. Line a couple of patty pans with the paste, and bake the tartlets until golden brown. Serve with vegetables.

EVE PUDDING.

1 teacupful of breadcrumbs, 1 small apple, peeled, cored, and chopped fine, ½ oz. citron peel chopped fine, 1 oz. sultanas, ½ oz. oiled butter, 1 egg well beaten, the juice and rind of a small half-lemon, sugar to taste, and a few finely chopped almonds. Mix all the ingredients, pour the mixture into a small buttered basin, cover and steam for 1 hour. Serve with sweet sauce.

No. 24.

MUSHROOM SOUP.

2 oz. mushrooms cut up small, ½ small onion chopped fine, 1 dessertspoonful of fine wheatmeal, pepper and salt, ½ oz. of butter, a little milk. Stew the mushrooms and onions together in the butter until well cooked, add ½ pint of water, and cook the vegetables for 10 minutes. Add seasoning, and the meal smoothed in a little milk. Let the soup thicken and boil up, and serve with sippets of toast.

BUTTER BEANS RISSOLES.

2 oz. butter beans, 1 tablespoonful of cold mashed potatoes, ½ small onion chopped fine, a pinch of herbs, ½ oz. of butter, seasoning to taste. Soak the beans in butter over night, fry the onion in the butter. Boil the beans in as much water as they absorb until quite tender. Then pass them through a nut-mill or mash them up, and mix with the fried onion, mashed potatoes, herbs, and seasoning; form into little rissoles, roll in breadcrumbs, place them on a buttered tin, place a few bits of butter on the top, and bake in the oven until a nice brown. Serve with vegetables.

RATAFIA CUSTARD.

½ pint hot milk, 1 egg well beaten, 1 oz. ratafia broken up, sugar and flavouring to taste. Mix the ingredients, pour the mixture into a small buttered pie-dish, and bake the custard in a moderate oven until set.

No. 25.

CLEAR SOUP WITH DROPPED DUMPLINGS.

Make ¾ pint of clear soup, and proceed for dumplings as follows: 1 egg, 1 tablespoonful of milk, 1 teaspoonful of fine wheatmeal. Beat up the egg, add the milk and smooth the meal with it, flavour with nutmeg. Gradually drop the mixture into the boiling soup, let cook for a minute, and serve.

SAVOURY SAUSAGES.

½ teacupful of breadcrumbs, 1 well-beaten egg, ½ teacupful cold lentil purée 1 small finely chopped onion tried brown. Mix the ingredients, adding seasoning. Form into sausages, roll them in a little wheatmeal, and bake them a nice brown in the oven. Serve with vegetables and sauce.

BAKED CUSTARD.

½ pint hot milk, 1 egg, a little sugar and flavouring. Beat the egg, mix it with the milk, sweeten and flavour to taste; pour the custard into a small pie-dish, and bake until set.

No. 26.

PARSNIP SOUP.

½ lb. parsnip, ¼ lb. potato, ½ small onion, ¼ oz. butter, pepper and salt, a little milk. Cut up the vegetables, cook them until tender, then rub through a sieve, return the mixture into a saucepan, add butter and seasoning, and as much milk as needed to make up the quantity of soup. Boil up and serve.

GROUND RICE CUTLETS.

2 oz. ground rice, 1 egg, ½ pint milk, a little nutmeg, a pinch of herbs, ½ oz. grated cheese, seasoning, and breadcrumbs. Boil the ground rice in the milk until stiff, add the egg, well beaten, and the other ingredients. Butter a flat tin and sprinkle with breadcrumbs, spread the mixture on the tin, sprinkle well with fine breadcrumbs, scatter bits of butter on the top, and bake until golden brown. Cut into pieces, dish up, and serve with vegetables and tomato sauce.

FRUIT TART.

Line a couple of patty pans with paste for short crust. Partly bake, then fill with any kind of stewed fruit, and finish baking. Serve hot or cold.

No. 27.

CHESTNUT SOUP.

½ lb. chestnuts, ½ small grated onion, pepper and salt to taste, ¼ oz. butter, ¼ pint milk, 1 teaspoonful of cornflour. Boil, peel, and mash the chestnuts, and set them over the fire with the onion, milk, ½ pint of water, and the butter. When it has boiled up, bind the soup with the cornflour, boil up, and serve.

MACARONI SAVOURY.

2 oz. of cold boiled macaroni cut small, ½ oz. grated cheese, 1 gill milk, 1 egg, 1 oz. fine wheatmeal, ½ oz. butter, seasoning to taste. Make a batter with the milk, egg, and meal, mix together with the macaroni, cheese, and the butter, previously oiled, season to taste; turn the mixture into a small pie-dish, and bake until a golden brown.

APPLE PUDDING.

½ lb. apples, 1 saltspoonful of cinnamon, sugar to taste, and some paste as for a short crust. Peel, core, and out up the apples. Line a pudding basin with paste, fill the basin with the apples, add sugar and cinnamon, cover with paste, and steam the pudding for 1 to 11/2 hours.

No. 28.

SEMOLINA SOUP.

½ gill of milk, 1 gill water, ½ oz. semolina, a very small piece of mace, ¼ oz. butter, ½ oz. grated cheese, pepper and salt to taste. Bring the milk and water to the boil with the mace, thicken with the semolina; cook gently for 10 minutes, remove the mace, add cheese, butter, and seasoning, and serve.

MACARONI CUTLETS.

2 oz. cold boiled macaroni, 1 egg, a pinch of herbs, halt a small grated onion, pepper and salt, breadcrumbs, and butter, or vege-butter. Beat the egg well, and mix it with the macaroni cut in small pieces. Add the herbs, onion, seasoning, and as much breadcrumb as needed to keep the mixture together. Shape

into cutlets, dip in egg and breadcrumb, and fry a nice brown. Serve with vegetables.

GOOSEBERRY POOL.

6 oz. gooseberries, 1 tablespoonful of cream, sugar to taste. Cook the goose-berries in ½ gill of water; when soft enough to pulp, add sugar to taste; rub the fruit through a sieve, let get cold, and mix the gooseberries with the cream. Serve with rusks.

No. 29.

CURRY RICE SOUP.

1 oz. rice, 1 pint milk and water (equal parts), 1 saltspoonful of curry, ¼ oz. butter, 1 oz. finely chopped onion, salt to taste. Cook the rice with the onion, curry, and seasoning in the milk and water, until the rice is quite tender; add the butter, and serve.

SWEET CORN AND TOMATOES.

1 teacupful of sweet corn, ½ teacupful tinned tomatoes, ½ oz. butter, seasoning to taste. Stew together, and serve with baked potatoes.

PUMPKIN TART.

¾ lb. pumpkin, juice of ½ a lemon, sugar to taste, some paste for short crust. Line a plate with paste. Meanwhile, stew the pumpkin, cut into dice, with a little water until tender. Add sugar and Lemon juice, and cover the paste, which should have been previously brushed over with white of egg, and bake the tart until the crust is done.

CELERY SOUP.

½ stick celery, ½ gill milk, 1 dessertspoonful of meal, pepper and salt, a little piece of butter. Cut the celery into pieces, set it over the fire with 4 pint of water, let it cook until quite tender, rub it through a sieve; return to the saucepan, add pepper and salt to taste; smooth the meal with part of the milk, add the rest and thicken the soup; boil it up for a few minutes before serving.

BEETROOT FRITTERS.

1 small beet, 1 egg, 2 tablespoonfuls of meal, 1 gill of milk, pepper and salt, a little Lemon juice. Cut the beetroot into small dice, make a batter with the milk, meal, and egg, mix the beet with it, adding seasoning to taste. Let some butter or oil boil in the frying-pan, drop the batter by spoonfuls into the boiling fat; fry a golden brown, and serve the fritters with vegetables and brown sauce.

BANANA PUDDING.

3 bananas, 1 gill of milk, 1 egg, a teaspoonful of lemon juice. Peel and slice the bananas, and cook in the milk until they will mash up well. Rub them through a sieve, add the egg, well beaten, and the lemon juice; pour the mixture into a small pie-dish, and bake in a moderate oven until the custard is set.

SANDWICHES

CHEESE SANDWICHES.

Cut some slices of rich cheese and place them between some slices of wholemeal bread and butter, like sandwiches. Put them on a plate in the oven, and when the bread is toasted serve on a napkin.

CREAM CHEESE SANDWICHES.

Spread some thin brown bread thickly with cream cheese, then put any kind of jam between the slices; sift with powdered sugar and serve.

CHOCOLATE SANDWICHES.

¼ pint cream, 2 bars of good chocolate. Grate the chocolate, whip the cream, adding a piece of vanilla ½ in. long; slit the latter and remove it when the cream is whipped firmly. Mix the chocolate with the cream and spread the mixture on thin slices of bread; make into sandwiches. If desired sweeter add a little sugar to the cream.

CURRY SANDWICHES.

Pound together the yolks of 8 hard-boiled eggs, a piece of butter the size of an egg, a little salt, a teaspoonful of curry powder, and a tablespoonful of fine breadcrumbs. Pound to a smooth paste and moisten with a little tarragon vinegar.

DEVONSHIRE SANDWICHES.

Cut some slices of new bread into squares, spread each piece with golden syrup and over this with clotted cream.

EGG AND TOMATO SANDWICHES.

2 eggs, ¼ lb. tomatoes, ½ oz. butter, pepper and salt. Skin and slice the tomatoes, melt the butter in a saucepan, add the tomatoes and pepper and salt to taste, and let them simmer for 10 minutes, mashing them well with a

wooden spoon; set the saucepan aside and allow the tomatoes to cool. Beat up the eggs, mix them with the tomatoes and stir the mixture well over the fire until it is well set, then turn it out and let it get cold; make into sandwiches in the usual way.

TOMATOES ON TOAST.

Cut in slices 1 or 2 ripe red tomatoes, after having removed the seeds. Arrange in a single layer in a baking tin, sprinkle with fine breadcrumbs seasoned with pepper and salt. Put a little bit of butter on each slice, bake 15 minutes, and serve on hot buttered toast; pour the gravy from it round the dish. A few drops of lemon juice are an improvement.